CHANGE YOUR MIND HEAL YOUR BODY

When modern medicine has no cure,
the answer lies within.

ANNA PARKINSON
Foreword by Benjamin Zephaniah

WATKINS PUBLISHING

LONDON

This edition first published in the UK and USA 2014 by
Watkins Publishing Limited
PO Box 883
Oxford, OX1 9PL
UK

A member of Osprey Group

For enquiries in the USA and Canada:
Osprey Publishing
PO Box 3985
New York, NY 10185-3985
Tel: (001) 212 753 4402
Email: info@ospreypublishing.com

1 3 5 7 9 10 8 6 4 2

Designed and typeset by JCS Publishing Services Ltd

Printed and bound by CPI Group (UK) Ltd, Croydon, CR0 4YY

A CIP record for this book is available from the British Library

ISBN: 978-1-78028-683-9

Watkins Publishing is supporting the Woodland Trust, the UK's leading
woodland conservation charity, by funding tree-planting initiatives and
woodland maintenance.

www.watkinspublishing.co.uk

Anna Parkinson is a former news and current affairs producer with the BBC. Her quest in 2002 to find a cure for her brain tumour led her to discover healing. She is now a practising healer and gives talks and workshops on traditional healing and natural remedies. She is also author of *Nature's Alchemist*, about 17th-century apothecary John Parkinson, who was herbalist to Charles I. She lives in Kent with her family. For more information see www.annaparkinson.com.

Contents

Publisher's note

The information in this book is not intended as a substitute for professional medical advice and treatment. If you are suffering from any medical conditions or health problems, it is recommended that you consult a medical professional before following any of the advice or practice suggested in this book. Watkins Publishing Limited, or any other persons who have been involved in working on this publication, cannot accept responsibility for any injuries or damage incurred as a result of following the information, exercises or therapeutic techniques contained in this book.

To my mother
with love and gratitude

Your stepping inwards from the air to earth
Winds round itself to meet the open sky
So vanishing becomes a second birth.
Farewell. Return. Farewell. Return again.
Here home and elsewhere share one mystery.
Here love and conscience sing the same refrain.
Here time leaps up and strikes eternity.

Sir Andrew Motion, 2006
Reproduced by kind permission of the poet.

Foreword

We all live in this modern world, dragging this body around town, doing stuff we should be doing, even though all the time we have this awareness in the back of our mind that there is something about this body we should know more about. There are aspects of our consciousness that were written about thousands of years ago. We get a glimpse of their power from time to time, but generally we stick with what's familiar to us today even though we yearn to know a bit more. Most of us don't know our own strength, but this story shows you how you can find yours.

I first met Anna as a typically conventional, educated middle-class English woman. She was informed, practical, busy, capable and sceptical, although she was always curious and open minded. Anna was a journalist, making radio documentaries for the BBC, and I was developing my poetry and writing novels, trying to get some unusual voices onto Radio 4.

This story begins some time after our paths separated. In the midst of her conventional life, Anna was hit with a diagnosis that would shake the foundations of anyone's world. She was told she had a brain tumour and learned soon afterwards that it was inoperable. You will read here the intensely personal story of how she battled to survive and emerged triumphant despite all the disappointments and disasters on the way. Eight years after the initial diagnosis, without any medical intervention, Anna's scan results showed that the tumour had shrunk to nothing more than a tiny piece of scar tissue, and if you met her today you would never guess she had been ill. As I read the ups and downs of her personal journey, which are sometimes sad, and sometimes funny, I feel the presence of an authentic voice which reminds me of who we are and what we can be.

Anna didn't go looking for this experience. She was just going about her life and it was suddenly thrust upon her. But faced with disaster, she explored and tested every possible solution, until at last she discovered healing. This book is the story of how she not only healed herself but became a healer. The remarkable thing about Anna's story is not so much her recovery as the discoveries she makes about the power of human consciousness along the way.

So many people have made claims for their power as healers and surrounded what they do with mystery. Anna demystifies the process of how healing works for anything from arthritis to cancer, believing that it is important to use your rational mind to help yourself heal. She shows us how ancient teachings and modern biological science correlate, explaining exactly why your mind has such a powerful effect on your body. It's Anna's contention that we all have the ability to be healers if we learn to listen to ourselves and use the power we have. She has mastered the art of 'going to the self of her self', drowning out the chatter and trusting the voice inside to lead her, and that is a journey of both power and mystery.

In a clear, accessible way she reminds us all how to breathe, how to love, how to live and the extraordinary things we can achieve if we trust our bodies, our selves.

Benjamin Zephaniah

Preface

In the summer of 1984 I was in Leh, the capital of Ladakh in northern India, interviewing the Dalai Lama. His visit to Ladakh that summer was a big event. Although it belongs to India, the Himalayan region of Ladakh is ethnically part of Tibet, and most of its inhabitants are Tibetan Buddhists. I had wanted to visit this place, sometimes known as 'Little Tibet', for a long time, to see what a Tibetan Buddhist culture would look like without the heavy-handed intervention of Chinese Communism.

Ladakh is mysteriously beautiful, albeit sparsely populated, poor and so cut off from Kashmir by the mass of the Himalayas that it is largely forgotten. That is why the Dalai Lama's visit was greeted with such excitement. The Ladakhis are devoted to him as their spiritual leader, and the spiritual part of their existence is deeply interwoven with their way of life. Some of their traditions exist for practical reasons. They practise a form of polyandry, for example. One woman marries several men in a family so as to keep the population down and eke out an existence on the precarious patches of soil that are not washed away down the mountains in the summer melt. But their spiritual practice is part of the daily rhythm of their lives. They prostrate themselves at the altars of the temples and shrines dotted around the country. They turn the great prayer wheels that surround the temple in the capital and murmur their prayers. Their devotion extends to sending away their young children to join the monasteries and nunneries that perch between the folds of the mountains, as Christians once did in Europe. In this way their children have a chance for spiritual education which, they firmly believe, brings blessings to all the family and the community at large.

The Ladakh capital fizzed with anticipation on the day the Dalai Lama arrived. The women's heavy headdresses were set with big lumps of turquoise. The monks stood out from the crowd in tall saffron hats. Strings of seed pearls, big hoop earrings, brown eyes and white-toothed smiles flashed in the sunlight. The Dalai Lama's party arrived in a cavalcade of open-topped jeeps, his entourage standing up in the back, like an army of holy bandits. There was a cacophony of welcoming noise from conch shells, trumpets and horns. Then, as the dust settled, a small man with an amused expression and an incongruous pair of glasses perched on his nose, stepped out to greet the crowd.

It had not been easy to arrange an interview with him. My formal letters and credentials from my employer, the BBC, elicited no more than a possibility. That possibility had to be negotiated in person right up to the day before the visit with the Indian official who was in charge of security. That's why, I suspect, there were no more than three reporters in the room when the time came for the Dalai Lama to give interviews, and all of us were young women. Any male reporter with the same intention was simply not equipped to give the Indian official what he hoped to extract as a price for his permission.

Whatever the reason, the three of us were hustled into a room so crowded with monks and electric fans that there was scarcely an inch of floor to be found. The Dalai Lama was seated calmly in a corner on the only chair in the room. The electric fans whirred noisily to keep a breeze going on his face and protect him from the stifling heat. There was nowhere to sit, and we could not stand in front of him, so we reporters knelt spontaneously at his feet, inches from his knees.

The BBC, where I worked, carries a status that makes this humble position unusual for an interviewer. I had tended to see myself as an equal of those I interviewed and often I was treated as though I was more than this. However, this interview was not a normal situation and the Dalai Lama himself was about to blow apart the ideas I had conceived about what was 'normal'.

I hadn't met the other reporters before but it turned out that we each neatly represented the culture that we came from. I was allowed to go first, and I introduced myself as 'from the BBC' and proceeded to engage His Holiness in a political dialogue about his position as temporal leader of Tibet. The BBC World Service, which this interview was for, talked about the world in terms of political divisions and the power of political leaders. I was thinking about my editors as I asked for the fans to be switched off so that they wouldn't interfere with the recording, and that only left me with

the worry of how these same editors would react to the
Dalai Lama's accented English, so I was determined to
get a clear statement from this interview that would be
politically significant.

The Dalai Lama, like most other Tibetan lamas,
has not been allowed to return to China or visit Tibet
since he fled in 1959, because he is held in such high
regard by Tibetans that the Chinese fear his presence
would incite rebellion. The Chinese government's
hope has been that the longer the lamas stay away, and
younger generations of Tibetans go through a Chinese
education, the fainter their attraction as spiritual or
temporal leaders will grow.

I had seen some evidence of this happening myself.
Between 1981 and 1983 I lived and worked in the
Chinese capital, Beijing. I was able to travel to most
parts of a country that was emerging from the vice-like
grip of Maoist doctrine, although I wasn't allowed to go
to Tibet. I had seen how religious sites and practices had
been stripped of their spiritual meaning. The temples
that had been reopened since the Cultural Revolution
were like painted museums for tourists and the 'monks'
in them employed by the state like caretakers. I had
been shopping in the city with one of the few Tibetan
lamas who was allowed to return to his people, the
tulku, Akong Rinpoche, and his niece, whom he had
brought with him from a visit to Tibet. He wanted to
buy her a traditional Tibetan costume for a formal
meeting with the Panchen Lama, a Tibetan spiritual
leader who had stayed in China under the 'protection'
of the Chinese government. But, try as he might, he

could not convince her to wear traditional costume. Her one desire was to possess a 'Mao suit', the matching blue jacket and trousers that were now beginning to be shaped and tailored as a concession to women's fashion, and this is what she ended up wearing.

So now I asked the Dalai Lama whether this 're-education' of the younger generations wouldn't make a permanent difference to the politics of his country, as the Chinese government hoped.

'What makes you think that the Tibetan people would want you back?' I believe I said. 'The younger generation have grown up in a different culture, so isn't there a chance that they would want to move away from the traditions of the past?'

His answer silenced me. He spoke a language like the wisdom of the oracle that I was too naïve to understand.

'When you are young, you see with one eye, and hear with one ear. When you grow up, then you see with both eyes and hear with both ears. So you see, what they think they want now may not be what they want in the long run.'

Was he talking to me or was he talking about the young Tibetans? I accepted his answer without understanding its personal implications for me while he turned to the next interviewer.

She was a young French woman from Radio France Inter. Her interest was the romance of the way in which the Dalai Lama and all Tibetan leaders before him had been 'recognized' in their infancy. Traditionally spiritual leaders perceive a new incarnation from signs in the actions of a baby. How could this system continue when the present Dalai Lama does not have access to the Tibetan people?

'When you die, how will they find the next incarnation? Will that be inside or outside Tibet?'

The Dalai Lama was happy to deal with that one. The situation has changed so perhaps the method of choosing a leader will change. It didn't seem to be very important to him.

'Perhaps they will just appoint a leader, or perhaps they will do as they do for the pope when the cardinals get together and see how the smoke rises from the room.'

Was he teasing us for treating Tibetan traditions as 'quaint' while we were happy to maintain our own? The Catholic Church has plenty of revered practices that predate the age of state government and democracy.

The last question came from the local reporter, a young woman from Radio Leh, and it took my breath away.

'Your Holiness,' she asked, 'can you explain please. Is the world an illusion, or the human mind?'

The Dalai Lama took the question smoothly, like the spiritual teacher he is.

'That's a bit complicated,' he said. 'The world is as it is. The question is how you perceive it. When you look to see where "I" is, you cannot find it. "I" is something relative. "I" exists only in relation to the world. So the notion of "I" is an illusion.'

I barely noticed this answer when he gave it. I was too busy marvelling at the possibility that this question and its answer were essential material for Radio Leh.

How would it be to live in a society where questions like this were routinely considered in public?

We were all speaking English – the Dalai Lama, Radio Leh, France Inter and I – and yet we were not speaking the same language at all. The only one of us who seemed able to master the experience of being human in all its forms was our interviewee. Every aspect of consciousness that we put before him was something he had considered. He patiently taught optimism, persistence and compassion, and has continued to do so for the quarter century or so since he gave that interview.

He believes that the truth of his message will become apparent to everyone in the long term, because it is based on the foundations of the human spirit. If humans don't cultivate their spiritual wealth as well as their material wealth they will come to realize some day that 'they have lost something very precious', he says. Eventually, in other words, the Dalai Lama believes that we all begin to 'see with two eyes and hear with two ears'. Since that interview, this has been my experience: the discovery of something very precious through facing the biggest challenge of my life. This book is the story of what I discovered.

Introduction:
One-eyed Vision

In the autumn of 2002 doctors discovered a brain tumour pressing on the right-hand branch of my carotid artery. That tumour and the symptoms it caused turned my life upside down and the struggle to overcome it was to be the greatest battle I had known. Yet, although it caused me pain and fear, and for a while cost me both my eyesight and my income, that tumour was the best thing that ever happened to me. It brought me insight into the true nature of my life. It showed me how to value and use what I have. It led me to understand my power as a human being. Above all it taught me how to love and be happy.

Many people say that illness gives them a new life. As the Dalai Lama says, 'Any tragedy forces you to re-examine reality and so it can be a good thing.' But if you are to enjoy the benefits of understanding that illness or disaster can bring you, you must first overcome it and return to health. This book has been written to help people who face major physical or emotional challenges do just that. I hope you will gain courage from my experiences and health from the methods I used.

In December 2010 I had what I expect to be my last MRI scan in a hospital for many years. It showed that what had once been a threatening tumour had shrunk to a negligible mass only 5 mm across – something akin to a memorial scar to remind me of what had once been such a significant event. I no longer have any of the painful and debilitating symptoms I once did and I am strong and healthy enough to do anything I choose. This change happened for me without any medical or surgical intervention because, I believe, I had changed my mind about how to live my life. Knowing how to live my life has saved my life.

I consider myself particularly lucky to have had this experience and yet I believe that we all have far greater power over the condition of our bodies than we imagine. I hope that reading this book will inspire you to develop your power to heal your own wounds. The tools I used and that I will explain in this book will help you to climb mountains in your life and assess the view from the top for yourself. Whatever I have done is within the scope of all of us and I trust this story will give you confidence in your power to heal.

I thought of calling this book 'How to talk to yourself', because useful introspection is a skill that most of us have lost. It is not valued in our culture, nor is it part of the habits of our elders as we grow up, as it once was. Nevertheless, it is, naturally, the quickest route to self-knowledge and, as such, the best way to understand our power in the world. The tools that you will discover here are ways to know the most important person in your life better, and that, whatever you may have been taught to believe, is you. When you know yourself better, you discover the paradox – that to know yourself is the best thing you can do, for yourself, and also for your loved ones. When you know what makes you happy and free yourself to create it, you are creating not just your happiness, but also your strength, and this is a benefit to those you love and to your community.

In pre-scientific cultures, from Africa to Hawaii, talking to yourself in one form or another has been the route to wisdom for hundreds of years. So the yogis and Buddhists have used meditation, while Africans, Native Americans and Aboriginals have called on spirits from ancestors, animals and the environment. When you use these old practices you recognize your harmony with 'external' forces at a deep level of your being. You develop a sense of unity and resonance with other beings that allows you to read them and gain strength from their ways. That sense of harmony, within yourself and with your environment, is beneficial for your body. The latest biological research confirms the beneficial effect of the old practices and gives a clear idea, for the logically minded, of how they might work. I believe this is important, because our mind, with all its power of logical deduction, can be our most powerful tool or our most powerful enemy. I will show you how I engaged my mind on my side, by feeding it with information that supported me in my quest for a happy, healthy life.

'Miracles' certainly happen. A miracle is merely a phenomenon that we can't explain and there are many aspects of life that no human being can explain.

The nature of life is more magic than most of us can conceive, and once you find one miracle, you begin to see them everywhere. But sometimes it's difficult to recognize the magic while you're going through it. This book will make it easier for you to recognize instantly the magic of your own life, and that is pure joy.

CHAPTER ONE

A Divine Joke

*I wanted to change the world. But I have found that
the only thing one can be sure of changing is oneself.*

Aldous Huxley, *Point Counter Point*

My mobile rings.

'Hello Anna. This is Ellen. Have you got a minute?'

I always have a *minute*.

'I just wanted to tell you that you've changed my life!
I'm pregnant and my man is totally committed to me.
He wants to marry me! And he has a new job with more
money. I'm so happy.'

I gave Ellen healing six months ago, and she had
phoned me a few weeks later to talk through a problem
she was having in her relationship. Now she's here
bubbling with joy.

'You know I've had therapy before but nothing
has changed my life like this has. I sing your praises
everywhere. I tell all my friends you're wonderful, but
you know that!'

I know what I do and I know how it can change
people's perspective, but the extraordinary things that

— 1 —

happen to them once they see things differently has little to do with me. It continues to amaze me.

I thank Ellen for giving me her news and go back to what I was doing before, feeling warm and encouraged and reflect on the conversation. I love what I do. When people thank me for a healing I find myself saying, 'It's a pleasure', using this stock phrase with genuine enthusiasm.

I never meant to become a healer. I didn't even believe in healing. But my body was my teacher. I found myself led into territory I had never previously considered, which changed my outlook on life completely. The external details of my life have remained much the same. I still live in the same house, love the same man, run or walk with the same dog. However, the view from the inside is radically different.

I would not have invited the experience I had, but through it I have discovered abilities that I dimly hoped existed somewhere but never believed that I possessed myself. In the process I discovered the profound abilities of every human being, with a clarity of understanding that has opened the door on mystery. It is as though I have climbed a mountain to see over the horizon and found a landscape that stretches endlessly onwards.

In the morning, I walk outside my back door and feel the thrill of the clear air on my face in the early spring sunshine. The air tickles my nose as it streams into my lungs and flows out again. I see a dew drop held in the crevice of a lupin leaf that sparkles like a diamond, and then I notice drops of the night's rain on every blade of glass, reflecting the morning light like a bed of seed pearls under my feet. Cowslips the colour of gold have triumphed over the bitter layer of snow and ice that covered them this winter, and the shriek of tumbling birdsongs tells me the other inhabitants of my garden are urgently engaged in the business of new life: finding fresh food, carrying moss to secret places and whistling their mates into line. Following their sound, I lift my eyes up to the infinite sky, where drifting puffs of mist float on the high wind. I am in paradise. Right here. Right now. My life is heaven.

As I walk, I'm aware how the bones and muscles of my foot fall gratefully into the soft turf. I feel the ground yield and gently push my foot back to me as I swing my weight to the other leg. My body is in charge of this operation. It knows how to balance the weight on one side to release the pulley of bones and muscles that swings my weight forward on the other. It's a small trick I learned over 50 years ago, but now I appreciate the *feeling* of it and the mastery of it in a way I never did before. If I had to calculate the path myself and co-ordinate the nerves and muscles perfectly I would be exhausted after ten steps. But my body never falters. I have learned to trust it, and to love it. It is my best friend. It cares more that I am happy than anyone else. When I am not happy, but only pretend to be, it is my body that protests and shows me where I have gone wrong. I love my body for that, and because it's the ship that allows me to navigate and explore this wonderful life.

OK, of course it's not every day that I'm so in love with life. Those are the good days – which are most days.

There are still days with frustration, when peace seems to have to be postponed, when my power is challenged and confidence needs to be restored. I still get myself tied up in plans made yesterday that I feel unable to change. Sometimes I feel a tightness in my thoughts and nothing goes right. I feel tempted to blame the person or the organization I am dealing with, the tool I'm working with, or my body for its limitations. But it's as they say: 'A bad workman blames his tools.' And I have learned to read the messages my body is sending me. I watch the signals and follow where they lead, understanding through them that my mind has been gradually creating a knot around me.

When I pause to reflect on the frustrations I am facing, it is as though I am having a conversation with the universe around me. Now I have understood this, I take time to find a solution to the problem that I am creating. I have learned to talk to myself. Paradoxically, that has shown me how to listen to the world around me.

I've read enough books on esoteric subjects to know that the author often describes having his or her spiritual insight since childhood. That was simply not true for me. I conformed perfectly well to the expectations of the society that I came from, and my spiritual self lay dormant until I was forced to explore it, in order, I believed, to save my life.

I grew up in London in an age of weak Christianity amid a stream of new religious teachings arriving from the East. The spread of Hinduism through the work of gurus with 'cult' followings was regarded with deep suspicion in the Western media, and stories abounded of sons and daughters who had been 'lost' to their families by transferring their allegiance to spiritual leaders.

My family's religion was established Anglican Christianity. One of my great uncles was a vicar and I used to sit in his Dorset church as a child, watching his formidable bald head bobbing above his dog collar like a cartoon bald eagle, counting the phrases that would lead eventually to freedom and fresh air. I was taught to pray to God on my knees before I went to bed. I uttered the words that I didn't understand and slipped under the covers with the distinct image of a white-bearded old man uncovering all my guilty secrets, peering at me through celestial floorboards as I lay in bed.

This was my idea of God. Christianity was associated with school and social acceptance. Until I was 16, I obediently went to church every Sunday at the insistence of my stepfather. No one ever asked me what I thought or how I felt about what I was hearing there. They would have been embarrassed by an open discussion about spiritual matters. As a young teenager I tried earnestly to put my faith in it. I was confirmed at the age of 14, in an absurdly short white dress, in the august atmosphere of the crypt of St Paul's Cathedral. After months of lessons aimed at making me truly comprehend Christianity, I still had the vague feeling that the teaching was as childish as my image of God peering through the floorboards. I felt nothing, and did not know where to go to understand God. The prayers I learned were remote and impersonal with no apparent effect, since we patently were not a society that promoted 'Peace on Earth'.

Such is usually the way with established religion. It becomes an organization that suppresses the individual, rather than enhances him or her, and this has a tragically weakening effect on our lives. We become powerful by association with the establishment – whether that is the Church, the government or the company. Establishments thrive on mass participation by individuals but they rely on conformity to their rules, and tend to be threatened by an individual's inspiration. To put it bluntly, we lose our souls by following the rules of society blindly, although we may gain success in social terms. We are trained from our earliest days to achieve this success, but it does not often make us happy. As Bertrand Russell said, 'Success is getting what you want. Happiness is wanting what you get.'

A few years later I let the Christianity of my childhood go and explored a different world. My elder brother went to live in a Tibetan Buddhist community in Scotland and in my father's eyes became one of the 'lost' ones. My mother's London home became briefly a staging post for visiting Tibetan lamas after my mother followed my brother into Buddhism and found herself a different Tibetan teacher. I was fascinated and delighted by the chance to get close to these teachers, but the images they brought with them seemed alien to my culture and threatened to annihilate everything I knew. I was repelled by some aspects I didn't understand, such as the pop-eyed black guardian deity, Mahakala, who glowered threateningly over a half skull he cradled in one of his hands. As far as I could tell, the message of Buddhism was that life was suffering, *samsara*, to be overcome by a process of withdrawal so that one could eventually reach the state beyond desire, or *nirvana*. I was fizzing with hunger to relish life. How could such a message appeal to me in my twenties?

Buddhism remained in the background for me because of my love for my brother and mother but I left all religions alone and concentrated on my life with energy. There were successes and failures. A degree in English from Cambridge, one failed career as an actress, one successful one as a BBC producer, one failed marriage, one successful one, two beautiful daughters ... and then, out of the blue, or so it seemed, something that changed my life completely – and taught me ultimately to understand myself as a spiritual being.

Few of us would bother to explore alternative ways of seeing reality if the one we experience on a daily basis were perfect. We expect to be happy, whether we consciously admit it or not. Our urge for survival drives us on, but so does our urge for happiness and comfort. We build families, homes, companies and cities in pursuit of this comfort and contentment. But when we are on the verge of losing it, when our bodies fail so that we risk never having it again, we realize that we have everything we need within our grasp all the time, if we just open our eyes to it. That is what happened to me.

CHAPTER TWO

Shocks and Surprises

Life is what happens when you're busy making other plans.

John Lennon

In that moment John Lennon sang the essence of our lives. Whatever our plans or skills, we are shaped by shocks and accidents that resonate with us at the deepest level of our souls. There is always a reason why what happens occurs, and it is a reason that is deeply personal to us, but often it's hard to see at the time.

Looking back I can see that one of the recurrent themes in my life has been the need to balance the relationship between male and female, in myself, and in the world around me. An individual, and a society, that balances the female, the emotional, receptive, nurturing part of consciousness, with the male active, creative will is healthy and happy. That has not been characteristic of Western society for hundreds of years, but I believe the urgency of waking up to the importance of nurturing our environment and ourselves is gradually creating deep changes. We know that we cannot sustain life from the unbalanced perspective that has built our wealthy society. We are rich but we are not happy. I believe we are now engaged in this kind of rebalancing and each of us has an important role to play in it.

The external details of my life have reflected this development. I was the youngest child born to a family of boys and to a mother who herself felt she would have been better loved if she had been a boy.

I was born in Singapore, the last of my mother's three children. My brothers were three and five years older than me. By the time I was born my mother's marriage to my father had limped into its final phase. He had left Burma, where I was conceived, to go to Djakarta – shortly to be the scene of the important Bandung conference that established the modern basis of power in Asia – in 1955. His work was important in the political scheme of things but shadowy, and he was not what he appeared to be.

Neither was his marriage to my mother what it appeared to be. We followed my father to Indonesia, where I was christened, but his secretary was already his constant companion there and my mother felt excluded. I was only two years old when she took us back to England on an Italian ship, filing for divorce soon after. This was the end of our little family, and my brothers and I grew up hungering for and idolizing my absent father.

We had an upbringing typical of an English middle-class family in those days. My brothers went to private prep schools where they were treated with mild brutality by war-damaged masters. I was kept at home and had a developing relationship with my mother and, four years later, my new stepfather.

My stepfather was a gentle and clever man but he didn't understand that children have feelings just like any adult. One evening when he sat in our sunny drawing room, my mother asked me casually if I liked him. I was embarrassed to be put on the spot in front of him. I thought he was astonishingly grey and as gloomy as a misty mountain. I later came to call him the 'marsh-wiggle' after the eternal pessimist creatures in one of C S Lewis' Narnia stories. However, as I had just been using his extra-long legs as a makeshift slide, and I was a polite child who didn't like to offend people, I said, 'Yes, of course.'

'Good, because I'm going to marry him.'

I was instantly happy to abandon my loyalty to my own almost-unknown father. I made an attempt to jump into the arms of this new dad. So it was a shock like the jolt from an electric fence when he put his long bony hands on my shoulders, and pinned me gently to the wall.

'I don't like small children,' he said softly, with a steely twinkle in his eye. 'I'm not going to be your father. You've already got one of those. I'm just going to marry your mother.'

He became a good friend to me and a good teacher as I grew up, but he never had to repeat his message that he would not be a source of paternal love.

As the youngest child, I sheltered with my mother while yearning to be part of the masculine world. I had very little success in my early years, when the masculine world consisted of my brothers' cricket team. My greatest success as 'deep fielder' was accidentally to stop the ball with my head from time to time.

However, as I grew older, my education and circumstances encouraged my unconscious desire to be recognized in a masculine world. I seemed to ride on the crest of a wave that other women had pioneered for me. Clare, my Cambridge college, had only been open to women for one of its 500 years of history when I applied for a place. When I graduated and went to work, I was the first generation of British women to benefit from the Equal Pay Act, which made it illegal to pay women less than men for the same job. In my working life, it quickly became clear that the environments that attracted me had been predominantly male preserves up to that point.

At first I pursued my passion for theatre, in Paris, London and New York. I joined a *commedia dell'arte* troupe, performing incongruously on the streets of Manhattan and the housing estates of Queens and Brooklyn. But I also found myself struggling with perpetual poverty and terrible temporary jobs so that, in the end, I decided to channel my passion for communication in the direction of the BBC. Eventually, I found myself turning up for my first day with the BBC World Service as a trainee producer.

Before I joined the BBC, I had no idea what a producer did, let alone how to do it. I had an idea that I wanted to give people a voice and help bring new ideas into being – as I was told this was what a producer did, I set about becoming one. It took me two or three years until I achieved my goal and when I finally found myself part of the staff, being given a tour of Bush House, where the BBC External Services were based in those days, it was as though the walls of Jericho had fallen. It was magical to find myself suddenly having access to information from all over the world, to talk to a correspondent almost anywhere at any time or read the tickertape machines from the Reuter and Associated Press news agencies running 24 hours a day. It was extraordinary to be able to go to a news library and call up well-organized back stories on any subject you could think of, so that you could give the impression that you had thought about nothing else for the last ten years. For someone more used to struggling street theatre performances, it was amazing to find that the words I wrote would be broadcast and listened to by thousands, perhaps millions of people across the world. This was 1983, when hardly anyone was using computers, and the internet was just a gleam in a few academics' eyes. In the days before Google, when information was preciously kept, working for the BBC gave you an astonishing feeling of having arrived at the heart of it all.

The Pursuit of Power

In the excitement and the headlong rush of work I was not aware of how much I had sacrificed to be there, nor would I become aware until my illness forced me to leave the BBC over 20 years later.

I focused my attention on news rather than arts, because I thought this would give me the best chance of securing a permanent job, so my love of poetry and stories was allowed to gather dust. At first I gave up regular sleep too, in favour of night shifts which entailed writing the news bulletin and producing the current affairs discussion programme at four in the morning – and woe betide you if you failed to understand the minutiae of Fijian politics at that hour. But there were other, more surprising, sacrifices that felt like I was being asked to change my values.

I went into the job as a believer in freedom and democracy, naïvely accepting that these were values the British establishment upheld. I had spent the previous two years, from 1981 to 1983, living in China, which was then emerging from the Cultural Revolution. The experience had been a fantastic political education for me, as I began to learn how an individual's life is shaped by the society he or she is born into. I saw how very different my outlook would have been if I had been born Chinese, as part of a predominantly peasant society, where starvation was a continuous possibility. I was proud of what I'd been able to learn there, and considered I had a valuable understanding of an important culture and language. My first job in radio was in fact for China National Radio, the international English-language service that was the Chinese equivalent of the BBC World Service.

I was astonished to find that I was rejected for a post I applied for in BBC World Service News because the editor considered me tainted by communist sympathies. He felt that having worked for the Chinese government editing in the Radio Features department,

I'd been complicit in creating propaganda. He was deaf to my protests that my job had been to filter out fantasy and insert truth where I could find it. As far as he was concerned I was a communist, and therefore unreliable. Little did he know that I had got the job in Chinese National radio by writing a play about the children's hero, 'Monkey', and getting the entire staff of the English-Language Features department to perform it!

After this incident, the role that the BBC World Service had to play in 'making everything in the UK garden sound rosy' grated on me. This function was one of the reasons that, unlike the rest of the BBC, which is funded directly from a compulsory television licence fee, the World Service was funded by the UK Foreign Office out of its own budget. Much as I loved the freedom of collecting interviews, crafting and mixing the recording tapes into interesting programmes, I could not get away from the fact that the news values were strongly biased in favour of showing Britain at its best. I soon moved off into what I felt was the serious world of news and journalism by going to work on the domestic news programme: Radio 4's *The World at One*.

My first morning on this job sent more naïve preconceptions crashing to the floor. When I walked into the production office at 7.30am to begin my first day, my heart sank, and I cursed myself for not having done a recce before accepting the job. There was a large table in the centre of the room, covered in editions of the day's newspapers, with a bank of telephone switch connections in the middle so that an incoming line could be answered by anyone around the table. Everyone there seemed to be dressed in grey suits, which I thought was odd since some of them were women. As the days went on I realized how unnecessary this formality was, as the pressure of putting the programme together to run at lunchtime that day meant that we hardly ever left the office. We could have had a uniform of bathrobes and bedroom slippers and it wouldn't have made much difference. However, the grey suit or its equivalent was the unstated uniform, and clearly designed to harness us all to the male corporate world. I once went in wearing a bright yellow dress and had to suffer continuous comments about my 'frock'!

The content of the daily programme would be directed by the editor, who would select the top stories of interest from the newspapers in front of him, as well as from the news diary that was prepared by the researchers. The opportunity to suggest stories would next pass around the table to the presenter and assistant editor, until finally it came to the newest and most junior producer to impress colleagues with an interesting and different idea. Clearly it was important where you sat on the table in the morning editorial round, otherwise you would be left with the very tail end of possibilities, but I was never much good at strategy. On the whole I was there to put orders into effect, however inane or impossible they sounded to me. Querying the editor's proposal was unpopular.

'I want Douglas Hurd on the phone now!' he would yell.

'But the Foreign Office has already told me that Douglas Hurd doesn't want to comment on this story.'

'Phone his personal secretary in the House of Commons and get him on the phone now.'

'The Foreign Secretary has made it perfectly clear this is not part of his area and he will not comment,' the personal secretary would say. 'What is the matter with you people when you can't understand a simple instruction?'

Enduring the humiliation of pressing for impossible results was a routine part of the news producer's life. This education in refusing to take 'No' for an answer would turn out to be a perfect preparation for my own personal battles that I could not have imagined at this stage of my life. Of course, that's not how I saw it at the time.

I felt bruised by the male misogyny of the place. It went deeper than grey suits at dawn. There were other women who worked there with me but if they weren't sleeping with the editor then I doubt they were any happier than I was. We all communicated in the harsh executive bark that was used on us when we arrived. We offered up stories that would be important in the political mainstream of the day; when I argued successfully for something different, such as a point of view from one of the Karen tribal leaders engaged in a 25-year civil war with the Burmese government, I was accused, to my astonishment, of having a 'penchant for little brown gentlemen'.

It was true, of course. I didn't want to join the others in the pub after work, where key decisions about the programme were made. I had no interest in making one of the editors or reporters my boyfriend. I was hungry for a broader view of the world. I was genuinely interested in the economic and social evolutions in south-east Asia, which seemed to me as important as the parochial interests of politics at home, so it became clear before too long that I was a fish out of water.

Nevertheless, the BBC was evolving under the influence of recruits like me, just as I was evolving under its influence, and most of my career at the BBC was not like this. I was able to move into a zone where I could make documentaries with and about people who interested me, and generally this involved showing the parts of the UK garden that were not smelling of roses but were in serious need of change. I was able to come up with ideas, persuade the BBC to commission them and then go out to meet and talk to people who I felt created change in our society by their thoughts and actions.

In the course of many years making those programmes a vital truth came home to me. This was that if you could get close to the source of a feeling, however humble, this would be an accurate representation of a greater economic or political reality. In other words, the macrocosm was in the microcosm. Many discussions about social and political affairs featured politicians who were studying the views of the 'experts' and the 'experts' were studying the actions and reactions of the people at the heart of the problem. It took just one 15-year-old girl and her friend to take it into their heads to go around threatening to stab strangers with an empty hypodermic needle – which could create an airlock in the bloodstream and so kill them – to create an entire social situation and generate hours of talk by people quite detached from their lives. What really mattered was how this girl and her friend *felt*. Their emotions about themselves, about their contact with strangers or with institutions, shaped society, whether they were aware of it or not. To be blunt, the only thing that would change the social and economic reality was the degree to which they felt loved or cared for. If you could change this, if you could make people happy, then you could change the situation they engendered and that would change everything.

But journalism could not change the situation. It could only reflect it. It held up a mirror to give people a voice, and sometimes the voice itself took over. People who needed society's attention would cast themselves in a role to get all the attention they wanted. They were just as likely, if not more likely, to get attention for creating damage and hurt around them as for creating good. Who ever heard of a programme about a peaceful and happy woman who was good at making her children feel loved?

My world was filled with clever people concerned about society and paid to change it, but who were unable to do so. We were journalists talking to politicians, who could talk about our society, like us, but were very rarely able to introduce a law that brought about the change they desired, and so very rarely able to tell the truth. There were economists, who would explain why the laws introduced by politicians had failed to achieve the desired results, being experts in retrospective commentary not prediction, and there were academics in the social sciences, who collected the views of people who created social and economic phenomena and relayed it to politicians and economists who were too busy to find it for themselves. Trying to penetrate this woolly world was a frustrating process and the frustration increased the longer you spent on the task, because the same stories came round again and again.

Once or twice there would be a 'big' story, exclusive information, which had the potential to create real change. I was given a story like this and I knew at once that it was the journalistic story of my career. Doctors in the big pharmaceutical department of a London hospital told me discreetly that they were under pressure to prescribe expensive 'named' anti-depressant drugs to patients in spite of the fact that they had found these drugs to be largely ineffective. Certainly they believed them to be no more effective than the far-cheaper unnamed generic version, and in some cases they were actively harmful. Considering that depression had become the third most commonly treated condition in the UK, this story had the potential to have a dramatic effect on NHS pharmacy bills and also to cast a searchlight on drug prescription in many other areas.

Delving a bit deeper it was clear that the trials which 'proved' the effectiveness of these drugs were seriously biased in favour of the drug manufacturer, a fact that very few prescribing doctors had the time or the energy to be aware of. My doctor sources were prepared to talk to me so long as they could remain anonymous – otherwise they felt that speaking out would cost them their jobs.

However, the BBC had just lost an embarrassingly expensive libel case to a drug company on a technicality. Try as I might, I could find no part of the corporation that was prepared to run my story. It was a question of timing, of course, or fate. The story did eventually run ten years later, but by that time my life had moved on. And for me this incident was the beginning of the end of my love affair with the BBC.

Powerless

The events of a beautiful autumn day in September 2001 were a dramatic reminder of the powerlessness of the powerful. They seemed to emphasize the hopelessness of relying on our institutions or governments to make our lives better. Like a brick thrown in a pond, they created turbulence and ripples that have since been felt throughout the planet.

I remember the clarity of the day. The air had crisped slightly with the end of summer, and the long cool night had warmed to the blazing blue of a clear noon sky. It was on a day like this that my first daughter was born, and I felt it giving me energy even on Oxford Street, where the buses and taxis lumber continuously by. Around 2.30pm I walked into Broadcasting House in London's Portland Place to have one of those prearranged discussions with my boss that you have when you are not quite sure where you are going next. I checked in with reception and waited for my meeting to begin.

I have always loved Broadcasting House. From the imposing curved front visible from the distance of

Oxford Circus, to the beautiful light frieze of Ariel carved by Eric Gill above its door, this building had come to feel as close as home and family over the years of intense work I had lavished there. My eldest daughter took her first steps in the marble reception hall, under the indulgent eye of her father and a BBC commissioner. I was upstairs in a recording studio at the time so I missed it all. I no longer worked there but I was always glad to have an excuse to revisit it. On this day I turned away from reception to glance at the television screens streaming the news. Out of a perfect blue sky on the screen was what looked like a toy plane heading directly into the recognizable twin towers of downtown Manhattan. As the plane collided with the middle of one of the towers it crumbled in a thick cloud of smoke. Both towers were melting under the open sky of this perfect American morning. -

The short burst of film ran over again and again. People entered Broadcasting House and stood like I was, rooted to the spot, everything else forgotten. Once glimpsed, this image changed everything. Could it be real, or was it someone's fantasy? We needed to know more. Again we watched, as the commentary and the terrified dust-choked faces of the people on the ground gradually brought home to us that something unthinkable had happened on a bright, beautiful morning in New York.

Journalists always feel responsible. They always feel that they must get involved whether they can do anything useful or not. If ever there was a big news story and we were broadcasting information as fast as we could get it, the broadcast studio would fill uncomfortably with the highest-paid news executives, still journalists at heart, all wanting to get their hands on the story and put their stamp on it. This event more than any other I remember was a call to action. The world was waiting to know who was responsible or how this had come about. It was clear to everyone that this was a decisive point in our history.

And yet for most of us there was nothing we could do – except watch and wait and claw over the strands of information that gradually emerged. We could review our ideas about Islam or American imperialism, or the role of Britain in international politics, but only a handful of people in the world could have prevented the escalation of this attack into the wars and deaths that have since ensued. When history is happening even the most powerful people in society feel powerless.

So where is our power as individuals? Does each of us have to be prime minister, or president of the United States, or a terrorist leader, to have an effect on the world? Even the people who reach those elevated roles are often driven by forces they can't control. Did the British prime minister have any choice about whether to support George Bush's plans for war on Iraq? If he had chosen not to support him America would have gone to war anyway. And if the president of the United States declared war on the Taliban in Afghanistan and Saddam Hussein in Iraq, did he do it because he felt that that was what an angry American public in his democratic country demanded of him? Would he not, as most leaders are, be damned if he did, and damned if he didn't?

The information revolution that has dominated our generation has added to this feeling of powerlessness. Ironically, at a time when knowledge has never been so easy to obtain, we grow further and further away from a sense of purpose and certainty. We get ever more intimate details of disastrous events in people's lives a long way away. The task of alleviating or preventing such distant disasters seems hopelessly daunting.

The American physicist William Pollard once wrote: 'Information is a source of learning, but unless it is organized, processed and available to the right people in a format for decision making it is a burden, not a benefit.'

The information that flows easily to us on a daily basis, through our televisions, radios and computer devices, has a physical effect on us. Momentarily, agonizing events from the streets of New York, the coasts of Japan or the Congo, become real in our living rooms. Our bodies go through the responses of compassion or fear, producing adrenaline to ready us for action that we will never take. However much we care, the task of reaching people thousands of miles away while we are occupied looking after ourselves and our loved ones is often insuperable.

The result is a slowly growing sense of powerlessness, as the scope of problems about which we are informed grows wider and wider. We are distracted by the lives of strangers whom we know more about than ourselves. What can we do that will make a real difference to the world? Can we even help ourselves?

Breathless

I certainly felt like this. In 2001 when the World Trade Center crumbled, the foundations of my own way of life were already shaky, although I wasn't aware of it. I spent my days in a frantic round of activity which brought me little satisfaction. I loved my family and my home, and I sometimes enjoyed my job, but I was aware of a black, untended chasm at the centre which was me. I spent no time paying attention to that.

I was informed but I felt ineffectual. As a journalist working in the news department of one of the most powerful media organizations in the world I was bombarded with information. But when a news story came up the odds of being in the right place at the right time to play a useful part in it were about as long as those of winning the lottery. I was no longer on the front line of news anyway. I made documentaries and that meant conceiving ideas and submitting them so that, even if they were accepted, they would only come to fruition perhaps a year later. It was a long and often dispiriting process and, despite my privileged job, I didn't feel able to express or explore journalism that was important to me any longer. I was almost perpetually frustrated.

On the other hand, I didn't feel free to walk out of my job either. I had a family at home who I was financially responsible for, and leaving my job would have meant selling our home to find a smaller one, with an uncertain future for our children. I felt profoundly stuck and I was looking for a way out.

We had moved out of London to a commutable distance when our children were very small, because we had no room in our flat in London and city life didn't seem to fit easily with children's activities. But now I divided my time in a breathless patchwork of trying to make motherhood and apple pie match a demanding full-time job in the city. I had been educated to think that a woman's work was worth as much as a man's. But I was finding that I longed to be a good mother on some forgotten level of my being, which was incompatible with wanting also to be a good and effective employee. I found it hard to enjoy satisfaction in either role.

My children knew where to find me when they wanted to ask me a question at home. I was always on the telephone or editing at the computer. At work I had my eyes on the clock and I was frantically trying to cram my tasks into the time I had available. I spent a lot of time running – never for pleasure – running for the train, or running for the bus to get to the train, or running to the car to get to the train on time. When work stopped in the evening or at the weekend I would cook or garden or build shelves, feeling that I was devoting what was left of my time to my family, but undoubtedly the work I was doing and its demands were always uppermost in my mind. The list of things that I gave myself to do each day left no room to feel or consider the really important emotional attachments of my life.

When my father was dying in 1995 I went to the house he shared with my stepmother, all of us expecting his end to come soon. He had been suffering from leukaemia for three years, and had grown painfully weak and thin. For the last three months he had been efficiently preparing for his departure and now we all knew that it was a matter of days away. Ironically, in death, if not in life, my father had all his children around him, except for my eldest brother who'd had to return to Australia. My father prepared to die like a Victorian patriarch.

The house was hushed when I got there. My exhausted stepmother and half-sister tiptoed carefully through the rooms. It felt as if we raised our voices or sat down too hard the household would break apart. My father lay upstairs in his bed. The rest of the family milled around downstairs, discreetly allowing one of us to slip upstairs and talk to him privately. He was hard to talk to.

When my father was still only 18 he had led a platoon of soldiers into Normandy as their extremely young and inexperienced captain. They were about three miles away from higher command and although they knew that they were to head north if the time came to retreat from the encroaching German army, they couldn't agree on which was the north star. My father made the wrong call. They went the wrong way. They were captured and he was to spend the next five years of his life in German prisoner-of-war camps. This experience had stayed with him for the whole of his life. We all knew how important it had been to him. He had an unspoken bond with fellow prisoners. His friends to the end of his life had all been prisoners with him, and yet it was an experience that none of his family could share with him. He was more comfortable with what he didn't say than what he did. For the rest of his professional life he specialized in official secrets, which we couldn't share with him either.

It seemed to me as though his romantic and family affairs stayed on a superficial level called 'normality', which even the greatest tumult could not break through. 'Normality' was never that in his life, but it could be managed so long as it was never emotional. While he lived I always felt that there was a barrier between us that I longed to break through, but to which I couldn't find the key.

When we were children, my father was almost a myth to my brothers and me. He was a brilliant but distant fantasy figure who we could never get close to. Once he sent a transistor radio to my brother at school. My brother would play it surreptitiously under the covers after lights out, feeling that by tuning into it he would hear my father's voice. His manner and appearance was like a real-life James Bond. Like James Bond he would appear out of nowhere in our lives after long absences, arrange to meet in anonymous places, like under the clock at Waterloo Station, drive us away in a sports car bearing the childish equivalent of champagne – armfuls of sweets. There were trips to the funfair, expeditions in a boat with just my father and us three small children as crew. Me so small, he said, that he had to tie me to the mast to stop me falling overboard.

I knew nothing about what he did, but I knew that when he was not with us in England, he lived in exotic places that our first memories had imprinted on our minds as delightfully warm and free of the censures that my mother's mother had introduced us to on our return to England. My mother did her best to maintain the curiously romantic dream of East–West bonding that we had been born into. We must have been the only children at the village fancy dress parties who turned up naked except for the grass skirts we had brought back with us from Burma. Our Burmese nanny came with us to English village life and sang me songs from the hit parade: 'Que sera sera' and 'How much is that doggy in the window?', which were the only songs I knew, well into adulthood. She sang the songs my father loved and I loved her with all my heart.

So my father was a mirage – remoter for me than for my brothers because he had never been there since my birth, and because when it was time to visit him in one of his exotic postings (it was Gibraltar – where my eldest brother was born – hardly exotic at all!) I wasn't allowed to go.

But he was a mirage that I loved. At the time of his death we had been able to talk to each other as adults for some time, but we had never broached that childhood chasm. I wanted desperately, as he lay dying, to be able to tell him how much I loved him. And yet as I sat upstairs by his bedside all I could say was: 'What are you thinking?'

And he said, 'Of all the things I can't do.'

Then I could only say, 'Would you like a glass of water?' when what I meant was: *I love you and I always have. I'm so proud of you – so glad to be your daughter – would you like a glass of water?*

Nevertheless, when my father died I began to discover things about myself that astonished me. First, that there was a kind of 'knowing' in me that was not dependent on words or facts. It was empathy, and I found it extraordinarily eloquent.

It was a state of communication that I had never previously considered. I knew exactly when my father was going to die – not to the precise hour, but which night it would happen. And I knew that he knew I knew. So we began to talk in a kind of code that he was comfortable with, from long years of professional experience.

I stayed the weekend, and then on Monday morning I went into his bedroom and told him I was going to work.

'How long will you be?' he asked.

Because I'm going to die today. I want you to be there and I can't hold on much longer.

'I've got a meeting this afternoon which is important, and I'll come back straight after that.'

Important??! Is a meeting with your colleagues at work really more important than being with your father when he dies?

'Well, don't be long then.'

I'll hold on till you get here.

'No, I won't, I promise.'

Message understood. I know you're going to die today and you'll wait until I get back. I'll be sure to be here. Thank you.

I came back after a day at work and my father was patiently waiting.

Around nine o'clock that evening he asked me to help him walk to the bathroom. It was a small request that had a powerful impact. As we staggered along the corridor together, I felt admiration for the dogged pride that forced him to get out of bed and use the bathroom as usual, when his weak body was so close to giving up forever. But I also took deep personal comfort from this little task. At last he was asking me for something he needed, and I understood his meaning: *I love you. I trust you and I know I can depend on you.*

Sad though it is that the culture I grew up in cannot express love, I felt this request was the closest my father could get.

At 2am that night he was sitting up in bed and his chest was rattling. We stood around him and watched him stare darkly inwards, helpless and breathless, until his spirit slipped away to another dimension.

Afterwards I lay back on my bed and closed my eyes. At once I found myself witnessing a dizzying battle between black and white forces in some unfamiliar cosmic theatre. I was fully awake, but the images in my mind's eye were as real as my physical surroundings. I was immersed in an unknown metaphysical reality that was communicating with me as clearly as if this was part of a continuing conversation that had been only briefly interrupted.

For what seemed a long time, the battle raged before my eyes. On the right side, jagged black-edged shapes morphed from witches to goblins while they fought the billowing clouds of white feathers and swirling streams of silver light that were ready to engulf them on my left. Back and forth this battle went and it was clear to me that I was witnessing a struggle in my father's soul, as though this was the most obvious thing in the world.

These black and white shapes seemed to me like the battle of fear and hope grabbing at him. On the one side desperation and despair drowned everything in darkness. On the other side, grace and eternal creation defeated the dark forces. I watched, transfixed by a level of experience I had never previously believed existed, until, at last, I fell asleep.

CHAPTER THREE

Even Doctors Pray

The feelings that my father's death stirred offered me a glimpse into a different way of seeing and understanding life, but the experience was quickly submerged under the sea of my daily activities. I returned to work and found myself, a few years later, moving away from producing documentaries to take up a managerial role. Ironically, considering that it was this event that had really brought home to me my lack of power as an individual, the role entailed co-ordinating a mix of archive material online to commemorate the first anniversary of the 9/11 attack on New York.

On 12 September 2002 I cleared my desk in Television Centre and prepared myself for an extended sabbatical that I had planned for many months. For some time I had been thinking about a book I wanted to write. One of my father's most precious possessions was a book published in 1629 by a family ancestor. He was John Parkinson who had been herbalist to Charles I, and this beautiful book, called *Paradisi in Sole Paradisus Terrestris* (Park in Sun's Earthly Paradise, in translation) was the first book about decorative gardening in English. I had been familiar with it all my life. My father had two copies and he would occasionally, in an expansive mood, slide one out of its hiding place and show off the elaborate woodcut of the Garden of Eden which was the frontispiece. My grandmother had made a gorgeous needlework copy of this woodcut which hung on my bedroom wall as a child. I knew its colours and its curious giant flowers intimately. But I had never actually read the book. It had always seemed to me that it belonged to a remote, antique world that could have no relevance for today.

However, when my father died I borrowed a copy from my stepmother and took the book home to read. I instantly fell in love with its author. He talked about plants that were familiar to me because I had been struggling to make a garden on several acres of untended Wealden clay that we had inherited with our house. But he spoke about the soil and the plants themselves with such a depth of understanding that his gentle wisdom leaped from the pages. It was like walking around my garden with the voice of ages whispering in my ear. When he talked about cyclamen, for example, he described not only its colour and form in minute detail, but also how it was grown in his garden and how to use the root and leaves for 'women in long and hard travels [labour], where there is danger, to accelerate the birth'. John Parkinson was an apothecary. He worked with plants, collected, grew, studied and wrote about them for most of his 83 years. He used his eyes instead of a microscope, his taste to understand the nature and the family of a plant, and his study, his friends and his experience to teach him how to use it.

When my second daughter was born in 1993 I had had 'long and hard travels'. I'd felt so exhausted by the time she was born that I'd had no energy to push her out. When she finally emerged, just before 4am on a Monday morning, the midwife tugged at the placenta and my womb filled with blood from the arteries that had fed it and would not close. I lay back in relief to be out of pain, while my blood drained away through the birth canal. Frantically, the doctors and nurses tried to pump new blood into my collapsing veins and get my womb to contract and seal off the arteries. Eventually, after passing eight pints of emergency blood through my veins, they told me they would have to remove the womb to tie off the arteries manually, and wheeled me into theatre to operate. But this was a teaching hospital and they were testing a new drug called 'Hemabate', which was intended for just this kind of haemorrhage. The senior registrar told me the next day, when I woke up in intensive care, that they had used this drug, and then, as a last resort, closed their eyes, crossed their fingers and prayed. Ten minutes later I stopped bleeding. I bless them for that and for their successful efforts to save my life and my womb. I remember feeling shocked that giving birth was still potentially so dangerous for women, and while I was thankful that my daughter had been born in hospital where fresh blood supplies and new drugs were on hand, incidents like this in my life began to develop my interest in the healing properties of plants.

I saw John Parkinson's knowledge as potentially practical today. His second book, published in 1640, described more than 3,000 plants and their medicinal uses. The *Theatrum Botanicum* (Theatre of Plants) was used as a text book by doctors and apothecaries for over 150 years. I wondered how someone who had contributed so much had come to be almost unknown compared to less-eminent contemporaries. Nicholas Culpeper, for example, lived through the English Civil War, like John Parkinson, and is popularly known today as a herbalist. However, his contemporaries had a low opinion of his skills, whereas John Parkinson was considered to be one of the greatest experts in Europe. I tried to find out more, but I was constantly confronted with the phrase, 'Not much is known about John Parkinson's life.'

This 17th-century apothecary's own story was a mystery. How did he come from nowhere to be the king's herbalist? Closer to home, was he, as my father had always maintained, a direct ancestor of mine?

I decided to write a book that would answer these questions and weave his life story into the stories of the plants that told so much about our ancestors from that time. Almost as soon as I had this idea on paper, it took off. A friend who I hadn't seen for years telephoned out of the blue. A professional writer himself, he was excited enough by my idea to give me some good advice and suggest I send it to his agent. She in turn gave me some more good advice, and within days I was steaming ahead putting together my book proposal.

So the letter that came from the hospital was an irritant. I dismissed the request that I present myself at the neurology department the following week as a distraction that would get in the way of the work I was at last able to spend time on. My husband, whose intuition is often sharper than mine, knew that something was up. I had had health problems intermittently for the past six years or so, starting, in fact, the year after my father died, but I had become expert at picking myself up and getting on with the job as soon as the crisis was over.

The first time it happened was the worst. In the autumn of 1996 I had been getting myself and my daughters dressed early one morning so that I could go to work and our au pair could give them breakfast and take them to school. My youngest, who was three at the time, urged me to put on (I mourn to say it) the white stilettos that she considered made Mummy look so beautiful. As I indulged her, I felt a crack across the back of my neck, like an axe hitting me at the base of the skull. The pain seared through me and I fell to my knees – where I stayed, only able to crawl to the loo and vomit water into the bowl. While I waited for the pain to subside, wave after agonizing wave racked my neck and body, as though my head was fixed in quite the wrong position. Our au pair arrived to find me rolling on the floor with just enough wit left to tell her where the doctor's phone number was.

I was still trying to work out whether I could get to work in time to go into the studio, where I was booked to record a programme, when my GP arrived, checked me over and called an ambulance. By the time I was in it, bracing myself in a lurching stretcher, my children were sitting in their classrooms at the village school listening to the sirens scream past.

That episode scared us all. I lay in hospital, in pain so intense that I couldn't sit up or eat, for five days while the doctors tried to decide what to do. They had a CT scanner, which they eventually used to produce multiple x-rays of my head, searching for an unusual bone or soft-tissue formation, but they couldn't see anything out of the ordinary in the dense tangle of tissue beneath my skull. They didn't have an MRI scanner, which uses magnetic resonance to make a more detailed distinction between different types of body tissue. If they had, perhaps they might have found the source of the problem. Instead they suggested I might have had a migraine and sent me home.

I knew this was no migraine: I had been an old friend of those in my teens and twenties. This headache laid me out for nearly three weeks. When the pain began to subside and I was able to move around again, every muscle in my body was sore and tender, as though someone had taken hold of my nervous system and put it through a mangle. However, once I was better, I went back to the life I considered 'normal', and didn't think about the incident again.

There were more episodes of the intense headache, which I came to recognize from the first second it announced itself. It always appeared out of the blue – often when I was feeling especially strong and healthy – and no matter how I tried to calm it, it always rendered me rigid with pain and I would end up in the back of the ambulance, on my way to hospital. But no one ever had an explanation, beyond telling me it was migraine. So I continued to ignore it.

I did try to calm down. I learned the Alexander Technique to try to ease out tensions in my neck and shoulders. My favourite position was a simple exercise I came to call the 'Fried Egg' because of the subtle sense of release that invaded my body when I remembered to do it – suddenly after ten minutes or so, I could feel the muscles in my back and shoulders spread out into the floor in a way that reminded me of a broken egg spreading in a frying pan. Lying on the floor with my knees bent and the tip of my head propped on a book, I could feel my neck muscles hang gratefully into the space I had created beneath them. The unfamiliar simplicity of merely watching my breath fill my chest, expand my abdomen and then drift into reverse was a pleasure. It was strangely fascinating to be so still for what seemed so long, and yet to watch the action in my body. My children loved to see me at floor level, a sleeping lion, and I could concentrate on this inner process even while they played and tumbled all over me. The calm this exercise generated proved to be infectious, so that if I lay on the floor like this after work, I could undo the ripples of tension in my body and also quieten my children ready for bed.

Even so, I found that I would ache when I got up in the morning, and I went to see my doctor. He declared it was 'old age', which shocked me enough in my mid-forties to make me resume a long-abandoned habit of doing a few yoga exercises every morning when I got up. That helped, and my children, who were used to a morning cuddle and my attention while they dressed and breakfasted, graciously allowed me my 'five minutes' peace' and adapted to the idea that I was to be left alone for that time.

I began to enjoy the unfamiliar sensation of carving out a space in my life that was just for me. I even cut down my hours at work for a while and did a part-time massage course. I wasn't sure why I was doing this, but it was a familiar pattern. Once before, I had turned to communication through a silent physical world when I felt unbalanced by too much mental activity: as soon as I had graduated with a degree in English literature, I had gone straight to Paris to study mime. Now I found that exploring massage revealed a similarly mysterious world and a much more subtle discovery of how the human body works than I had imagined.

On one level I was enjoying rediscovering how the muscles and the organs function, revising for the anatomy and physiology exams that were a requirement for the course by drawing out the muscles in blue felt-tip pen on my children's wonderful bodies. On another level, the practice of massage revealed an exchange of something between humans that fascinated me.

People would get up from the massage table delighting in their bodies, feeling soothed and energized. Often they would say, 'But you must feel so tired!' I would check and discover that it was the opposite. Concentrating on giving people energy gave me energy and made me feel better than before. Energy – what were the properties of this curious sensation that was so vital and yet didn't appear in any of the medical text books? How had it been overlooked? Why did my doctor never mention it?

Once, the art of massage, or 'rubbing' as it was called, was considered an essential part of a doctor's art. Hippocrates, the Greek doctor whose oath to medicine is still sworn by every graduating doctor, taught that: 'The physician must be experienced in many things, but assuredly also in rubbing; for things that have the same name have not always the same effects' (Aphorisms of Hippocrates, 460–380 BC).

He was talking about what the fingers 'read' when they touch another body. The benefits of massage, described in physical terms, are that it stimulates the immune system and encourages cells to release excess uric acid into the bloodstream. Even a novice masseur can perceive this happening under the skin, but this in itself is not enough to account for the profound effects that massage can have. I was beginning to discover that my fingers could sense a volume of information when I touched another body with the intention of making that person feel better, and I was curious to discover more of what was to me then an uncharted world.

These activities opened a 'valve' in my life that I felt allowed me to breathe, but sadly none of them could touch the demon headache when it reared its head. Another physical problem was beginning to emerge. I found that my eyes would lose focus if I sat and looked at something for a long while. When my husband and I went to a play that had two people on stage in the first act, by the second act I would see four. I began to go for tests at the local eye hospital, but no one could point to a cause.

So when the letter arrived from the neurology department in September 2002, I was perfectly used to hospital appointments and not unduly bothered. I had gone for an MRI scan a couple of weeks after the most recent headache episode but I assumed that the deterioration in my eyesight had something to do with that old refrain: 'middle age'. Certainly I was wholly unprepared for what happened when my husband and I walked in to see the neurologist together.

'Take a seat.'

We sat down side by side, as before the headmaster's desk. He leaned back in his chair and fixed his eyes on me.

'You've got a brain tumour and it's going to have to come out.'

I felt myself melt into the plastic seat.

'How?'

'Well they cut along the side of your nose and they can go in that way. After a few years you can hardly see the scar. Or else they take the top of your skull off, lift the brain aside and go in that way.'

Silence. I mentally picked myself off the floor.

'When?'

'Oh, in two or three months.'

'What happens next?'

'We'll be in touch.'

We staggered out.

Perhaps it didn't happen like that. Perhaps the neurologist explained carefully what the implications of such a surgery would be, how it related to the problems I'd been having with headaches and my eyes, but I don't remember it like that. What I remember is that we went home, stunned into silence, and immediately hit the internet to try and get some idea what was going on.

When the neurologist said they would be in touch, he meant, of course, when the laboriously slow process of letters and referrals to a neurosurgeon at another hospital had taken its course. This meant three months before I would see a surgeon who would tell me exactly what they proposed to do.

An appointment in three months gave me plenty of time to panic. Of course I didn't know what the statistical likelihood that I would go blind or die was, but at the time I felt it was the sort of information that would be helpful. We tried to find out more but I didn't even know what kind of tumour I had and my husband and I were soon to discover a dazzling variety of names and experiences of brain tumours. But I knew one thing with crystal clarity straight away – if I was going to go blind or die, I was damn well going to finish the book I had started first.

So I quickly settled into a pattern where I would work feverishly on my book during the day and wake up in fear and trembling about 3am every night. The work I was doing felt like a blessed escape from having to think about what was happening to my body, but I couldn't really get away. Nothing could touch the loneliness and fear of those night hours. It was always a relief to see the daylight.

At the time, it was the surgery that scared me most, not the potentially fatal end result of having a tumour in the brain. Yet it never occurred to me that I could make a choice about what was to happen to my body. The doctors seemed to have ultimate authority. The British National Health Service is a wonderful institution, which delivered my babies and has patched me up after many disasters in the past. However, every good thing contains its opposite, and the downside of our universally free British National Health Service is that we deliver our bodies to a doctor at the first sign of illness and assume that it is up to them to 'take care of it'. The more serious the diagnosis, the more inclined we are to leave it entirely in the hands of our doctors to sort out. The extended Latin names that they use to describe each new condition – like *fibromyalgia* (pain in the muscles) or *meningioma* (an unspecified growth of tissue in the brain lining) make our sick bodies sound too technical for anything other than a specialist to be able to understand.

I certainly fell into that category. If they had told me I needed to have my eye removed in the first weeks after the diagnosis, I would simply have made a date in my diary for the procedure to take place. An arm or a leg? Of course. Which one do you want? In the vacuum of information and the months of nightmares that followed that first visit to the neurologist, I was only concerned with finding a doctor who could remove the problem from me and do as little damage as possible in the process. Nevertheless, there was a refrain going through my head, like a stuck record, playing out as I walked with my dog across the fields, in imaginary conversations with the doctors I had met. It went like this: *Be careful. This is my head we're talking about. It may be just a case to you, but I've only got one of these and it's very precious to me!*

When I met a doctor who was overly business-like or failed to meet my insatiable need for information, the refrain shrieked at me for days afterwards, but I wasn't in the habit of really listening to myself and I carried on doggedly consulting doctors and trying to decide what to make of the information they gave me.

I was extremely lucky in two respects. Thanks to my stepbrother, who is a doctor, I was able to find the man who was recommended as 'the neurosurgeon doctors would choose to go to'. I was referred to Michael Powell, the specialist surgeon in pituitary tumours at the National Hospital for Neurology and Neurosurgery in Queen's Square in London. Michael Powell has a broad, bald forehead, gold-rimmed glasses, a genial smile and patience you could fry an egg on. His staff adore him, and I had been told by an enthusiastic radiographer on my first visit that people came from all over the world to see him. He brushed aside the scans I brought with me from the other hospital as 'too poor quality to be useful'. He was confident that once he had good-quality scans he would be able to excise the problem and my life would go back to normal.

I felt as though I had met a man who I could trust to understand my feelings, though I could barely express them because I didn't understand them myself. The second great stroke of luck, which I didn't recognize as such at the time, also stemmed from Michael Powell becoming the surgeon in charge of my case. He is a cautious man who wanted to solve the problem for me, but after his initial optimism that the tumour would succumb to his skilled knife, he eventually said he couldn't operate.

The tumour was growing with the right-hand branch of my carotid artery wrapped around it. Given the pressure of blood pumping through the carotid artery and the mass of nerves that surround it, this is not an area that a surgeon wants to go near.

So, not only was he reluctant to operate, but he was equally reluctant to go in to collect a sample for biopsy, to see if the tumour was cancerous. It was too deep, too difficult to get at and, if it was cancerous, there was a danger that puncturing it would spread cancerous cells to other parts of the brain.

In fact, once he and his team had studied scans showing the size, position and behaviour of this tumour in my head, he was able to tell me . . . nothing. They didn't know what it was.

'Ninety-five per cent of pituitary tumours are just that. Then there's four per cent that are something else (information the doctors give you passes swiftly by!) and the remaining one per cent is made up of about 150 types. Yours is one of those.'

So after all the panic and the nightmares, I was now in a position of 'waiting to see'. I wasn't quite sure what we were waiting to see. Presumably we were waiting for the tumour to grow so fast or its effects to become so crippling that removing it would be worth the damage that surgery was likely to do to me.

Every few months I would go to London for an MRI. For 45 minutes I would lie in the scanner, not daring to move a muscle, while what sounded like a crowd of weird monsters drilled through my head. By the time they had finished with me I always felt that it was only a matter of time before they would have to cut my head open, and of course, that would be the end of life as I knew it. I would dry my tears in the square outside and stagger to the nearest café to cheer myself up. Then, a few weeks later, I would go to the hospital, filled with anticipation, to see the results. In the early days my husband came with me, because I felt I wouldn't remember what they said to me at this all-important meeting. We would be shown into a roomful of people. These were all specialists in different disciplines studying the 'case'. Michael Powell would diligently and kindly introduce each of them in turn until I was mystified about which one to talk to. I would throw out the symptoms I had been experiencing like fish into the sea, and someone would swoop and swallow each one. It was civilized, genteel and maddening.

'I've been exhausted so I can hardly get out of bed in the morning and my period has lasted for three weeks. Could that be related to the pituitary?'

'It happens at your age,' said one of the wise gentlemen. 'We call it menstrual chaos.'

We all laughed and nodded.

It's all very well for you! I seethed inwardly.

This process went on for months. No one wanted it to be a great drama, no one wanted an emergency operation, but meanwhile I could feel my life falling apart. Then, as sometimes happens with our National Health Service, it descended into chaos.

I sat in the hospital waiting system filled with a familiar feeling of anxiety mixed with anticipation. I watched the line move from the outer room of the hospital department where I was seen, ever closer to the doctors' consulting rooms. Hospital waiting systems are fascinating in their way. I became quite an expert in those years. You can't predict how fast the queue will move exactly. Each cluster of people is there for a different doctor or set of doctors, and they may be patients or they may be companions. So you can entertain yourself with a guessing game of matching patient to consultant. It's a difficult game to win, because, as we all know, people are not what they appear to be.

On this occasion I moved from the outer hall to the inner corridor and then things seemed to grind to a halt. Patients who appeared to be 'behind' me went ahead, and medical assistants came twice to check my name and hospital number with me. At one point Michael Powell left the consulting room and returned about ten minutes later.

Eventually I was shown into his room. The doctors and specialists were arranged around the room in their familiar semicircle, with Michael Powell sitting behind the desk like the chief spider, wearing a benignly puzzled expression.

'This is very embarrassing,' he said straight away. 'We can't tell you anything about the result of your most recent scan because we appear to have lost the scans.'

At that time the scans were produced as large x-ray sheets, nearly two foot square, with multiple images on each one, produced in a series which showed the object being scanned from fractionally different angles. The number of images was almost overkill, but no images at all, well . . .

He went on apologetically.

'I've been up there myself to check, but your scans have been mislaid, and we have nothing at all we can show you.' In consolation, he offered, 'This has never happened before in all the years I've been a consultant.'

So I grinned bravely and left with my tail between my legs. But all the way home I was thinking: *Why me? Why does this unprecedented event have to happen to me? Why do I have to have something that they can't diagnose, can't predict the behaviour of and, right now, can't even scan?!*

They had promised to call me in as soon as they found the images, but this turned out not to be so easy. Once they appeared to have located the problem and found the notes and the images from my MRI, I took the precaution of getting copies of both notes and scans, and began to send them off to get opinions from other doctors. My stepbrother had recommended a radiologist in Seattle to me, and he had also heard good reports of a neurosurgeon in San Francisco. I sent these doctors copies of my records to see whether they thought they could do anything for me.

They certainly could, they said. The radiologist from Seattle said the tumour was cancerous, but he could destroy it using new gamma knife laser technology alongside his PET scanner, which uses radioactive signals to take precise images of functioning parts of the body. The neurosurgeon from California agreed that it was a *chondrosarcoma* (cancer) but nothing else. He trusted to his traditional surgical skills and said he would be able to cut the tumour out with his knife. Meanwhile I had also sent the images to a neurosurgeon in Paris recommended by another friend. The view from France was that it would be best to leave it alone, to 'wait and see'.

I was spinning in a world of mystery. The experts' opinions cancelled each other out, which made them as good as useless. Which one to pick? Not only was the nature of the tumour itself unclear, but there seemed to be new techniques for attacking it springing up all the time. There were very few surgeons in the world using gamma knife radiation with a PET scan at that time, though my research uncovered one in Bologna. This was almost home territory, and I might even be able to get the treatment on the National Health Service, since it wasn't yet available in the UK. Briefly, I pictured myself enjoying a luxurious Italian holiday, with a short intermission in an Italian hospital while a surgeon blasted laser rays into the deepest part of my brain. On reflection, I hesitated. Paris and London had agreed on a 'wait and see' policy. Reluctantly, I decided to go with this and stay at home.

'Waiting to see' involved regular trips to the hospital over the next three years to lie in a scanner or perform increasingly impossible eye tests to check the range and function of my right eye. It involved living with a bucket-load of symptoms that left me feeling weary and depressed. I would wake with the impression that an elephant was sitting on my head, or not sleep at all. Some days my energy would be 'normal'. Other days I was so dizzy all day I felt sick. When I was feeling energetic I was liable to be struck down by a sudden headache that arrived without warning. Eighteen months after I was diagnosed, I recorded one of these events in my diary:

About 4pm on Saturday I was digging and bending over to pull out roots and stones when I suddenly became aware that I had a pain right across my head. I recognized the pain and thought I had better stop immediately. By the time I'd kicked off my boots and got inside I could hardly walk because it got worse so quickly. I tried to lay my head on a book, Alexander Technique style, and rest my shoulders on the floor – but the book hurt my head too much. I was incredibly hot and suffocated and then I began to get cold. I couldn't find a position to rest my head in and I took two Migraleve tablets. Clara [my daughter] helped me to bed. She got a bucket in case I was sick and a hot-water bottle because by that time I was freezing cold. The tablets eased my pain after half an hour, so that I could stop crying and writhing and rubbing my head and at least talk to her. Then about an hour and a half later the pain started to come back again – like ripples of fire and ice breaking open my head, in spasms so I couldn't lie still.

The effects of these episodes lasted for over a week and the impact on my family was devastating. Everyone was tense and argumentative. We all found things wrong with each other. On top of the effect on my energy, the impact of the tumour wasn't pretty. My right eye slowly drifted inwards as the tumour pressed on the nerve that controlled its outer muscle.

I was beginning to study anatomy in far greater detail than I had ever needed to before. The way my eyes were *supposed* to function became intensely interesting to me. I was surprised to find that the mechanism that controls the movement of the eye is apparently simple, considering the complexity of information decoded at the back of the retina. There is a muscle either side that moves the eye from left to right, like a horse's rein or a pulley, and a muscle above and below that moves the eyeball up and down. In addition there are two muscles that wrap around the circumference of the eye ball. Basically these six muscles allow you to move the eye to any position to the front or side, but they also adjust the focus of your sight. When the circumference muscles are taut with tension, the round shape of the eyeball is compressed and lengthened, so that the distance between the lens and the retina grows. In this state, objects far away will seem fuzzy and unclear because the lens projects the image just short of the retina. If this is habitual for you, then you are called short-sighted. When the muscles that move the eye from side to side and up or down, the rectus muscles, are over-taut, the round shape of the eye ball is flattened. Objects close by will seem unclear because the distance between lens and retina is too short and the point of focus is just behind the retina. This is what we call farsightedness.

But there are also other ways in which the muscles around the eyes can go off balance. Tension on one side of the body or another will show in one eye only so that the sight is uneven (astigmatism) or one eye will seem to be 'lazy', allowing the other one to do all the work of focusing and processing information, while not co-ordinating with it. I now looked as if I had been cross-eyed from birth. My right eye was pointed permanently at the bridge of my nose. However, I soon discovered that understanding the muscular mechanism of the eye wasn't much help to me. The tumour had 'palsied' or paralysed the nerve that controlled the outer rectus muscle. It was as if I had dropped the reins on the right and the nerve in charge had become like worn elastic. I would have to go deeper to find a solution to the problem.

I wore a patch on my stronger eye and tried to 'exercise' the soggy right one. I was using my eyes intensely every day, to research and write my book, so the 'patch' treatment (which I had devised myself as a possible way of bringing my right eye back to life) exhausted me. The ophthalmologists at the hospital pointed out that when my right eye was focusing in front of me, my left eye was working overtime underneath the patch. So every time my right eye was in the centre, my left eye was looking to the extreme right to get the right one into position. Naturally, this was exhausting.

So I gave up and left off the patch except when I was driving, when I covered up the weak eye. The DVLA took my driving licence away and replaced it with a temporary three-year permit. I began to feel I was going rapidly downhill.

The hospital ophthalmologists eventually proposed a Botox injection to try to correct my eyesight for me.

Botox is a toxin that paralyses the muscles. It's used as a beauty treatment because muscles that have become accustomed to tensing with anxiety in the forehead are unable to do so once they're injected with Botox. In fact they're unable to do anything at all for about six or nine weeks, until the effect of the Botox wears off.

They injected Botox into the inner muscle that controlled my right eye, the 'left-hand rein' as it were, to paralyse it so that it wouldn't pull the weakened 'outer rein' so strongly. The right amount of Botox, in the right place, would, they calculated, allow my right eyeball to return to centre.

The injection into the muscle behind my eye was intensely painful, despite local anaesthetic, but mercifully short.

'Did you feel any pain?' the surgeon asked afterwards. He had carefully applied the anaesthetic and gently used an electronic pulse to monitor the exact destination of the Botox.

'Like 30-second childbirth,' I said, through gritted teeth.

He looked a bit dismayed. He had taken so much care to avoid pain, but of course a local anaesthetic doesn't reach that deep, and he didn't understand what I was referring to anyway.

However, the effects of this injection were delightful. When I took the bandages off a couple of days later, I was exhilarated to be able to see everything clearly. I had got accustomed to my new way of seeing the world, and even found advantages in it. The dislocation in my eyes meant that I could look from two angles at once, so

I often had the impression of seeing someone coming before they actually arrived. I found the sensation that I could see 'around corners' quite interesting. But to have my eyes restored to crystal clarity was intoxicating. My energy shot through the roof.

Except that this wonderful effect soon wore off. Like a 'perm' or champagne, the world seemed so much dimmer than before when the old reality returned. The eye surgeon tried to repeat his first success a couple more times. But he couldn't get the position exactly right again. There was either not quite enough toxin, so the eye was still pointing inwards though not quite so much, or the toxin leaked into one of the muscles that control the up and down movement of the eye, so that my right eye was permanently raised heavenwards, in mock astonishment.

'They say the first time is always the best,' said the surgeon ruefully in his gentle Irish lilt. 'Like champagne. It's never so good as the first time.'

In the case of my eyes, a miss was as good as a mile. A little bit of double vision was even more difficult to cope with than a lot. So we left off the Botox and the patches and I resigned myself to having one eye, effectively, while we carried on 'waiting to see' how the brain tumour would develop. Until we could establish what the tumour was, what its progress was likely to be and what could be done about it, nothing could be done to help me. In the summer of 2004, the 'wait and see' policy descended into farce.

On 1 June my husband and I went to the hospital for the result of a scan that had been done a fortnight before. I had begun to lose my faith in these visits. They had once seemed so important and decisive, but I now expected little from them. That didn't stop me from being disappointed when we were shown in to see the consultant and his team.

Technological advances in surgery were moving so fast that we had found there was now a neuroradiologist in London offering the gamma knife treatment that I had considered in Seattle or Bologna. We were curious to know whether my consultant thought that this approach might suit my case.

'We have your scans this time,' he said, smiling with relief.

He listened to the question about referral to the neuroradiologist we'd identified.

'Yes, of course I know his work and I would be happy to refer you to him. Unfortunately there is still a problem. We haven't been able to locate your previous scans, so I have nothing to compare these results with. I'm afraid we can't give you any conclusions from this set of scans at all and I won't be able to refer you until we find them.'

'I have copies of the earlier scans. I could have brought them with me if you'd let me know.'

'Yes, well, unfortunately we weren't aware of this problem until about half an hour ago, so I'm afraid we'll just have to carry on looking and discuss the images when we find them. You won't need to come in again. We'll let you know.'

We went away for a week's holiday on a leaky boat on the Norfolk Broads. It seemed entirely appropriate that

I should spend my fiftieth birthday floating around in circles between the reed beds.

'They call them the "Broads"', my husband said, 'because all the people on the boats are broad.'

We watched another case of beer disappear down the hatch of the boat moored next to us.

CHAPTER FOUR

Intuition as Inspiration

You are not alone. Just your idea of you is alone and that is an illusion.

His Holiness the Dalai Lama

There was an undercurrent bubbling along meanwhile in the depths of my life, but so far down in the murky water of my mind that I was only dimly aware of it. I had managed to give myself a daily discipline, grateful for the breathing space it gave me, the sense of existing for myself. Every morning, before I had time to talk myself out of it or think of doing anything else, I would spend about five minutes doing a few yoga exercises and then sit cross-legged on the floor, close my eyes and breathe.

In the beginning, I wasn't sure what I was looking for. I knew only that I wanted space, and the only place in my life that I could find it was inside. At first I would sit in a half-lotus position, the yoga position where you bend one leg in so it rests on the floor at the base of your body and you cross the other one over it. Gradually, as this became comfortable and easy to do, I would try a full-lotus position for a bit. Each leg is crossed onto the other thigh and the legs seem to make an intricate knot that supports your body. It was hard to do at first and my legs would cramp after about ten minutes, but I persisted. I adopted this position in the interests of balance. With my right eye refusing to co-ordinate with the left one, it seemed important to me to use every means I could of balancing the two sides of my body. But the position had another significance for me that made me stick it out.

My family had 'form' with yoga. My mother's father had a good friend who had published a book about yoga for the British public in 1937, *Yoga Explained* by Francis Yeats-Brown. The physical exercises made such an impression on my grandfather that well into old age he used to stand on his head for five minutes every day, allowing the MCC striped tie that he favoured (Marylebone Cricket Club, for the uninitiated – whose home ground is Lords), drape in front of his face. As a small child I admired this mild eccentricity. His bald head made me think he must be at least 100 years old.

However, when my grandfather tried to teach *me* how to do a lotus position, I couldn't do it. My legs didn't seem long enough to make any kind of knot and when I crossed one foot on top of the other thigh the other foot would fall out.

After a few minutes my grandfather gave up.

'If you can't do it now at the age of three then you'll never be able to do it!'

This hit home. I already knew that as a girl I was considered no use on the cricket field. It was the word 'never' that got to me as a three year old. Now, here I was, in middle age, still trying to prove my grandfather wrong. Not *never*, but in my own time. In fact, I don't think it matters what position you adopt for meditation to start with, so long as you're sitting up and you don't fall asleep!

I was familiar with yoga movements, or *asanas*, but meditation had somehow eluded me for a long time. My earliest experience of meditation was as a 15 year old growing up in the heart of the hippy explosion that had overtaken the King's Road in London. In the district so poetically called 'The World's End' where I lived, there was a kind of drop-in centre where meditation sessions and talks were held every Wednesday evening. I used to go occasionally with a school friend. It felt edgy and we enjoyed being welcomed into what seemed like a secret underground group, although the meditations we all did together were long and we had no idea what was going on. Later, as a 20-year-old student in Cambridge, I inquired about learning transcendental meditation. I discovered that it was necessary to bring an offering and make a vow of obedience to a picture of a guru at a ceremony overseen by a white-robed Englishman with a beard. I balked. The school friend who had explored the World's End meditation sessions with me had by this time gone to live in a commune off the Irish coast with the father of her four-year-old daughter. This wasn't the lifestyle I had in mind for myself and making obeisance to an unknown guru seemed to me somehow dangerously close to it.

Later I learned some meditation techniques from my mother's Tibetan teacher, Lama Chime Rinpoche. In my early thirties, I was going through a considerable amount of pain with the collapse of my first marriage. I asked him to teach me. I was surprised to find him reluctant.

'You're too young,' he said. 'You've got other things to do.'

Eventually, when I persisted, he taught me a couple of mantras, sacred sounds (which I didn't know the meaning of), to repeat over and over again. I tried this for a while, confused about what was supposed to be happening, and then abandoned it. So he was right: I wasn't ready, and I did have other things to think about.

Now I decided to try again. But how to begin?

The yogi science of breathing, or *pranayama*, has a breath exercise for every imaginable physical state – and some unimaginable ones too, like being buried alive for hours at a time without oxygen. I wasn't sure that I could see the point of this, but this was the stage in my life where I stopped needing to know the point before I did anything. I was so worried and confused that I stopped using my mind and just did the thing. Once I determined to look for strength in the only place left available – inside – I discovered that the only thing that had been lacking before was my determination. Now, imperceptibly, I had begun a journey. I decided to start very simply.

I would sit in a half lotus, close my eyes and breathe. Paying attention to what I was doing, I took a deep breath and let the air stream out of my nose for twice as long as it took to take the next breath in. Then I did it again. I set myself a goal to spend at least ten minutes doing this every day, without expectation, concentrating only on the rolling continuity of the breathing. I was just breathing, not relaxing my muscles or looking for any other achievement. Easy. It felt pleasant. I was learning to be still. To enjoy my body.

As I watched my breathing I became aware of being a physical channel between the earth and the sky. I was feeling the process of oxygen streaming into my lungs from the air around me to animate the solid form of my body. My body felt like the earth itself, delivering spent energy as carbon dioxide to the grateful plants on the planet. If I could, I would sit in my garden, surrounded by grass and trees, and imagine myself in conversation with them, yielding the gas they needed for their growth while they gave me mine. It felt like being an essential cog in a turning world. It gave me strength and solidity. For those ten minutes, my mind was at rest.

Once I had begun this practice, I was reluctant to give it up. I found I could squeeze in the time by getting up earlier, or sometimes I could do it on the train. I was aware of the conversations around me, and realized that the lives people were talking about reflected the life I had been leading.

'He does nothing but work. Ted came in one morning and found him asleep at his desk. He hadn't been home all night.'

'She doesn't care. She's got the kids and the horses and the house. She stays at home and spends the money.'

'Sometimes I open the fridge in the kitchen at home and I think, "Who eats all this food?" I pay for it but I'm never at home to eat a meal. It feels like I'm just there to pay the bills.'

I listened to these conversations with mixed feelings of identification and detachment. I could see myself in any one of these people, and yet I had the feeling that there was another conversation going on in me that sounded different. It had a profound, solid, reassuring feel about it – like a beacon that guided me through the thousands of things a day that I felt I should do but didn't necessarily want to. Like a torch guiding me out of a thick wood. This conversation came from those few minutes a day I spent watching my breath.

At the time I was making some programmes about puzzles and how people solve them. One of our interviewees was British mathematician, Andrew Wiles, who had distinguished himself by finding a solution to Fermat's last theorem, a mathematical puzzle that had been unsolved for more than three and a half centuries. I know nothing about mathematics, and I don't even understand the purpose of the theorem, but to mathematicians Fermat's last theorem was a potentially beautiful creation, awaiting only the mathematical proof to make it complete. Andrew Wiles told us that he worked on finding a way to prove the theorem every day for 12 years. I was struck by the visual world his description of thinking the problem through to its solution evoked. He said that every day he would go up to his workroom and go over the work he had done the day before.

At the beginning, you go inside [your mind], and the room is all dark. You're stumbling about and you have no idea where you are. Then you begin to detect some pieces of furniture in the room and you become aware of where they are. When you visit again you know they are there and can begin to see how they relate to each other, and the details gradually become clearer and sharper. Then suddenly one day you go in and all the lights come on, and you see the whole room lit up!

In fact, when Andrew first published his proof, some fellow mathematicians pointed out a flaw in it. He and his assistant devoted a further two years to the problem before they repaired the mistake and came up with the solution that has been universally accepted. From which you might conclude that the most valuable tool we have to uncover the power of our minds is persistence. I was just beginning to glimpse the continent within.

When I closed my eyes and watched my breathing, I became aware of my body from a new perspective. The view from inside felt quite different from what I was accustomed to. I watched my mind travel to dark spots, to places where I felt pain or tension, and as I became aware of these places from the inside, it was as though I became the owner of them. I began to feel in charge of my body and its feelings for the first time. Just to be aware that I felt tension in my neck or my hip was powerful enough for me then to be able to decide to let it go. Sometimes it worked instantly. Sometimes it didn't. But the possibility of directing the internal traffic was there, and this gave me a sense of strength that I had lacked before when I felt buffeted by the incessant waves of daily activity around me.

So when the devastating diagnosis of September 2002 arrived, I was already slightly familiar with my own inner weaponry. This didn't prevent the symptoms from appearing, nor did it stop me falling headlong into fear and confusion in subsequent months. But I didn't stop meditating. When I was ill, I knew that I needed it more than ever.

Sometimes words came up that seemed important, so I recorded them. Three months after I was diagnosed, during a time when I was haunted by nightmares, I wrote this in my diary, without knowing what it meant or where it came from:

The solution to the problem is in the person
Find the person who's in charge of the problem. Is it you?
Put the person in the place where the problem can be solved
Starting on the thin ice of truth.
When the person is in the right place the problem will go.
Pop! The balloon will burst.

Was it a poem or was it a prophecy? I had no idea. In fact it would be two years before I understood what these words meant and how they could help me out of my predicament. They came out of the deep subterranean territory that was part of my whole being, and part of every being. It was territory I knew very little about, but which I was about to have to explore. The fact is, I would eventually discover, as my favourite

Hawaiian, Harry Uhane Jim, says, 'You don't know all of you, but all of you knows you.'

After my diagnosis, I realized there was an urgent need to learn the language of this subterranean territory. Damien Hirst has described the place where 'the impossibility of death in the mind of someone living' meets 'the unyielding reality of human decay' as the place of Ultimate Reckoning. The sense of Ultimate Reckoning within me was creating vibrations at the deepest level of my being. In my conscious state, I had registered that death might occur sooner than I had anticipated, but I was too busy to think about it. My husband and children did me the favour of appearing to pay no attention to my squinting eyes, headaches and dizzy spells while I carried on writing, cooking the dinner and taking the children to the normal round of school, theatre classes and dancing lessons.

The nights were a different country, though. My dreams were pitching me into fearful situations that I had to struggle to escape.

I was standing outside a huge stately home that seemed to promise a perfect way of life. Its French windows opening onto a graceful terrace were inviting, but then I looked more closely and saw that the windows were boarded up and the brickwork was crumbling. All along the terrace were cracked washbasins that had been hastily erected as a makeshift bathroom for the inhabitants. I wasn't supposed to enjoy this house any more. I was one of the refugees milling around on the terrace outside . . . not allowed in.

I was stuffing myself into an underground train with a lot of other people who wanted to get on. I pushed through barriers and then discovered I was stuck in the top part of the carriage, unable to stand up, crawling on the shoulders of people beneath me, unable to breathe or see or get anywhere.

Then I was driving in a red car that belonged to someone else around a walled city, trying to get in. We came to a gate in the wall and tried to drive in, but the arch was so low that the car got stuck and wouldn't go inside.

I was travelling across the world in an aeroplane, trying to land in Geneva in Switzerland. But the plane landed in Basle and there was a mountain to cross to get me to where I needed to be, or another plane to find and that would be hard. I was angry. The people who booked my ticket had done this deliberately, leaving me stranded in the mountains.

I was strapped into an old-fashioned perambulator, swaddled in blankets so I couldn't move my arms or legs. It was a dark, rain-swept night in the city, and someone had left me on a hillside. The pram was hurtling down the hill towards a black lake. There was no one in control. No one to stop me. No one to hear me. Help! Wake up please . . .

I awoke feeling dazed and confused. It became hard to get to sleep at night. I took herbal remedies like valerian or melissa before bed in an attempt to make myself drowsy. Often they had no effect and I was awake all night. Then the next night I would sleep heavily and wake suddenly at 3.30 or 4am, desperate not to sleep any longer! My dreams became as real as my waking thoughts and yet I had no idea what was going on.

My own mind was speaking to me in symbols and parables which I didn't understand. I decided to pay proper attention. I became intensely interested in myths, legends and totems, which seemed to be already familiar to my subconscious self. Gradually I pieced together the language I was dreaming, to discover a different sort of language from the one I was used to.

Dreams are the place where our unconscious selves emerge most naturally, especially when we are under stress. The subconscious mind, I found, makes no distinction between physical and emotional reality and ignores the limitations of geographical space or linear time. So our dreams can tell us far more than we consciously know, if we pay attention to them. I found my dreams effortlessly reaching to the place that my conscious mind could not yet go: that part of my self which is, in essence, also the universal source or fabric of the universe.

Sometimes dreams can be prophetic, since they allow you to look at your experience from a perspective that is greater than the one you habitually use in your waking state. The more you trust the power of your intuition, the more you will be able to understand this prophetic guidance when you need it. Lama Chime Rinpoche tells the story of escaping from the Chinese soldiers over the Himalayas into Nepal after the Chinese invasion of Tibet in 1959. He was the abbot of his monastery in Kham at the time, but he was also just 16. As he fled with a group of monks across the mountains, he dreamed one night that the Chinese would appear ahead of them and cut off their path. When he woke he told the monks that they would have to go back the way they had come and take another path, but they didn't believe him. They thought they would be returning into the hands of the Chinese army. Eventually he persuaded them and they later discovered that if they had stayed on their original path, they would certainly have been captured. After this, whenever they were lost, or there was a doubt about which way to go, they made Lama Chime take a rest and guide them with his dreams.

Dreams incorporate all the paraphernalia of our present lives but they are also a profound reflection of ourselves seen from a grand perspective. When we can understand them, we are beginning to take stock of our position so that we can guide ourselves more easily in the direction we want to travel. The truth about our dreams is the truth about our lives also.

I began to remember my dreams and record them as soon as I was conscious, by talking about them or scribbling the details in a notebook. My husband would listen tolerantly to crazy stories in the morning, with no apparent reaction. He maintained that he 'didn't dream', meaning only that he never remembered his dreams when he awoke and saw no reason to try. For me, however, dreams had become the opening scenes in a fascinating conversation I was beginning to have with *myself*.

I understood that my dreams were showing me my deepest feelings. This meant that the most important aspect of them to remember when I began to consider them later in the day was *the way I had felt* about what was happening in the dream. My dreams were expressing feelings that I had not been giving myself permission to feel in my waking life. Clearly, when I dreamed of being squeezed into an underground train or stuffed into a pram that was hurtling towards a black lake, my dreams expressed my fear at being engulfed by a chaotic situation that threatened everything I loved and seemed to me beyond my control.

I learned to understand my dreams with the knowledge that *everything in my dream was me*. The cars or the houses or the trains I dreamed of were my body, the 'vehicle' where my soul lived. The shape or form that vehicle took in my dream told me something about what I felt about that body or where I thought it was going. Even when I was dreaming of loved ones or enemies or colleagues, I was dreaming about a part of myself. There was an aspect of that person that represented my image of myself, or a role I had taken on, which needed my attention.

As I began to unravel my dreams I was impressed by the gravity of the mind that was unveiled in my sleep. It drew my attention to the seriousness of the situation I was in, which my conscious mind preferred to gloss over or seek distractions from. And yet, while every emotion appeared as an object to my night-time self, I could in my dream somehow engage with things that, awake, I found overwhelming. Interpreting my dreams, I found I was watching fear fearlessly, and it was immensely soothing.

As I began to understand what my dreams were telling me, the frequency and the ferocity of my nightmares diminished. The night-time language began to change. Dark, confused landscapes, littered with debris, gave way gradually to a brighter, more colourful world that enriched my days. Horses, birds or fish spoke to me. I discovered the universal dream language, which is different from any other. It moves simply but swiftly from the technical to the primeval and embraces an understanding that dazzles the conscious mind. Dream-time intuition is linked through symbols that we subconsciously understand to distant cultures like the Mayans, the Cherokee or the Zulus. It expresses the evolving state of your 21st-century consciousness with reference to experiences far removed from your own. It expresses something you know before you are told, which is, nevertheless, the voice you need to hear today.

I began to get a sense of knowing by the answering echo of my intuition when a definition or description of the meaning of what I had dreamed was the right one for me. My subconscious mind was telling me truth and it was a voice I no longer wanted to avoid. I was beginning to feel I had an inner guide to take me forward, and it was talking in my sleep.

Your dreams are where your personality and your Spirit are in contact, giving you information.

Martin Brofman

This is a record from my diary of one of my dreams and how I interpreted its messages to guide me:

Summer Solstice 21.06.06

I dreamed I walked into a clearing and there were people there, dressed in soft loose robes. They were guides who had a message for me which was that more pyramids had been discovered and I needed to see them. They pointed me in the right direction and I thanked them and rode off that way. I was aware that I had been frightened of horses before and never truly been comfortable riding one, so I was nervous and wondered if I could ride well enough. I know also that the horse is me. In Chinese astrology I am a wooden horse, so riding a horse is coming to terms with myself and accepting my nature. For the Native American shamans it was the spirit of the horse that enabled them to travel to the inner realms. Riding the horse in my dream was like flying, galloping with smooth confident leaps I had never experienced before. The horse and I were one because I loved the horse and trusted him completely, just as I love my faithful sheepdog, Benjy.

We galloped through a glade of trees and as I ducked under their sweet branches, I was aware that they were birch trees. Birch trees are hardy northern forest trees that give a sweet wine made from their sap, a protective oil and a preservative can be made from their bark, as well as them being traditionally used to sweep away rubbish or inflict punishment because of their strong flexible branches. These trees were often used to make canoes in northern Europe also and this is an analogy I often use as the vehicle of your journey through this life. When your mother and father come together and create your life, it is as though they give you a canoe and a paddle which is yours to steer as you wish. You can stop where you like and guide the canoe to any destination you choose but it helps to be aware of the flow of the water (emotion) in which you are living so you do not get stuck by trying to paddle upstream.

The fresh green glade of trees in my dream was a passage through love to the other side, sustaining and feeding me on my journey. I was aware that these trees were feeding me oxygen, and nourished by the carbon dioxide that I and my horse expelled as we swept forward on our quest.

On the other side I was surprised to find a busy village with more guides who had just time to tell me that I needed to go underground to find the pyramids. I was surprised that I had to go down to find these undiscovered symbols of unity and wisdom, but that is the nature of travelling into the subconscious. I went down to the very basement and found myself looking onto a field of tiny sparkling pyramids, each one made from the deepest lapis lazuli. Lapis lazuli is the blue stone used since ancient times as a pigment to create the blue of the Madonna's robe. The deep blue of the sea and the sky represent the subconscious and the conscious mind respectively, and blue can also be the colour of healing and mystical perceptions.

The pyramids were laid out on a grid and at the side of the field there was a man poring over a model of them trying to work out a pattern or break a code. It was as though he was working on a circuit board, and trying to make the connection that would bring light. While he was doing this there was a woman next to me who was shouting at him, suggesting he was stupid for not seeing how simple and obvious the key to the grid is. I was caught between these two, with the man on my left and the woman on my right, but of course they are both me. The masculine aspect of myself is trying to work out the map and the method precisely. The feminine aspect of myself is bossily and rudely pointing out that the male can't see the wood for the trees and he's making it too complicated.

We haven't yet reached unity. That is still to come. I need to calm down the impatient female and look more closely at the minutiae the man is studying, allowing her overview to guide me so I do not get lost. That is for a meditation or another journey in the night.

CHAPTER FIVE

Meditation as Medication

Heaven Earth and I are living together, and all things and I form an inseparable unity.

Confucius or Chuang Tse,
Chinese philosopher, 4th century BC

While my dreams were still turbulent, detailed and disturbing, the meditation I had begun to do daily was, by contrast, a calm and simple process which became more and more important to me. It was a vital sanctuary and a therapeutic tool: indeed, the only one I had at my disposal. My husband, with his usual sharp instinct, began to refer to the time when I would take myself off and shut out the world for half an hour as my 'medication'. And so it proved to be.

The months after my diagnosis were like sailing in a wildly stormy sea, and I found my life perpetually astonishing. Ways in which I had felt perfectly in control of my daily reality seemed to slip through my fingers. It was as though I had been adding 2 + 2 since the day I was born and suddenly I was finding that the answer was 5. My dreams reflected that sense of being carried somewhere by a vehicle I could not master, but at first they seemed a part of my imaginary world and not reality as I knew it. I thought I could escape from them when I was not actually sleeping.

What surprised me most was not *my* emotional reaction to the situation but the unpredictable emotions of my loved ones. Friends and more distant family were concerned and sympathetic, making a special effort to telephone and stay in touch with what was going on for me. Meanwhile those who I lived with began to behave in a way that seemed more than I could cope with. Was it really reasonable of my husband to check through my emails and throw a hissy fit over an innocuous message to a long-time ex-boyfriend? Was this really sufficient grounds for separation? Did my mother *have* to phone and ask me to drive 16 miles so I could help her get her earrings out of her ears? And did my daughter, who I had always considered clever and trustworthy, really have to destroy her grade card and forge a new one so that her grades would look better than they were?

It didn't take a genius to realize that the emotional temperature in the household was running danger-ously high and something needed to be done about it. I was familiar with using the tool of argument and persuasion, but that quickly met its nemesis in the form of my mother and my husband, either of whom would continue to return an argument to the point of mutual distraction or else apply a deep freeze to the whole matter.

It wasn't completely clear to me then that this state of domestic turmoil had anything to do with me or my illness, but I knew that it was eating me alive. I was tortured with guilt and anger in addition to trying to cope with the symptoms of my illness and finish the task of writing my book, which was an opportunity I had hungered for and the one achievement I wanted to complete.

Matters came to a head one summer day in 2003. The catalyst for what became a profound rearrangement of my life and relationships was my mother, appropriately enough, since she brought me into the world. We had had a testy relationship for some time. My brothers had lived abroad for many years. But although my husband and I had chosen to live close to her, eight miles from her house in Kent, I found her demanding and insensitive to my needs and problems. She was dealing with difficulties in her own life, because my stepfather – her husband now for over 40 years – had developed Alzheimer's and become almost completely dependent on her presence. My mother regarded me as her back-up in this situation, and I accepted this, but resented the fact that my efforts were taken for granted. On top of this she reacted fiercely to any sign of dissent from me.

When I told her my initial diagnosis, she barely responded. It was as though she couldn't quite take the news in. A month or so later she suggested that I take on the job of organizing an eightieth birthday party for her.

'I think you should do it. You're good at organizing things, and you should have plenty of time now you're not working.'

I didn't want to agree. But I didn't have the sense to say no. As the weeks went on the difficult balance between us, over who decided what for her party, became increasingly tense. The whole affair made the minutiae of every decision she had to make my responsibility, and my resentment increased. I asked her not to ring me so often. Surely once a day would be enough. So when my brother and his family arrived from Australia for the party, she stopped talking to me completely.

My brother would ring instead: 'Mum says, have you arranged to collect the glasses because she knows someone who says they will deliver them?'

I took my children round to her house to spend time with her and their cousins. They went off to the garden studio while I went into the house to say goodbye to my mother. As I stepped in through the back door she appeared. She jabbed me sharply in the middle of the chest, pushing me back the way I had come.

'I don't know what you're doing here.' Jab. 'You don't want to be here anyway.' Jab. 'So go on. Get out. Go home.' Jab. Jab.

Furious at being pushed out of her house, full of resentment at her unequal treatment of me and my brothers, I pushed her back. I'm taller than my mother, who is small and thin, and, you will remember, was then nearly eighty – an indomitable spirit in a fragile body – so when I pushed her, she fell sprawling on the floor.

Luckily she was unhurt, but my guilt and shame were overwhelming. Like red-hot pokers I felt them burn in me, and I decided enough was enough. I knew that if I was to have any hope of survival I would need to deal with this much raw emotion. I was angry with my mother for taking up all my time and I was spending more time being angry with her than I was doing anything useful for her. This kind of waste had to stop. As I was also still experiencing days when my energy seemed suddenly to fall through the floor, I needed to conserve all I could.

But how to resolve it? Any discussion with my mother was out of the question. I had tried in the past to explain my feelings to her and each time it had ended with her tears and even greater frustration on my part. In the end I was forced to reach out into the unseen world of energy and discover that trusting in *that* world changed everything.

I understood very little about the concept of energy then. Apparently my doctors didn't either, since they never had any suggestions when I asked for help, but I knew that the absence of energy was a living death. But I had begun to read widely: the kind of books I wasn't accustomed to, books like this one, which offered me a way to get out of my difficulties. I was reading books about feelings, books about energy and *chakras*, books about faith and books about angels. I read hungrily, without prejudice, although sometimes I wrapped a book in newspaper, furtively wishing to conceal its contents from strangers.

I was beginning to get a picture of the ancient wisdom that perceived a connection between the living energy of human beings and the energy inherent in all other matter. By developing the ability to still their bodies and their minds to very deep levels of awareness, teachers of the past became sensitive to minute variations in energy.

Communication by means of energetic signals is apparent everywhere in the animal world and human beings are no different in their ability to detect and understand energy. It's a faculty we all possess but which we have almost forgotten how to access. In the modern 'civilized' world we have obscured our understanding behind verbal communication, confusing ourselves in the process. We regard ourselves as important minds with a body attached, rather than as thinking animals. We allow our instinctive faculty to perceive energy to be overrun by learned rational thinking. However, what we say is often not what we mean.

To understand what we know and what we can do we need to learn first how to resist distraction and focus on internal signals. Individuals from earlier cultures, who could do this to a very great degree, gradually developed charts of energy flows in the body that have become a guide for the less intuitive modern world. For the Chinese, energy in the human body flowed in 13 pathways from the crown of the head to the soles of the feet, called *meridians*. For the yogis of India, energy flowed in three pathways interlacing the spinal column, called *nadis*, and collected in different densities throughout the body in seven levels known as *chakras*. The ancient Hawaiians, whose healing philosophy has a beautiful simplicity and logic to it, talked of three centres of energy along the spine, at the level of the navel, the solar plexus and the crown of the head. They called these the child, the mother and the father respectively, explaining their interaction in a way that must certainly have inspired Carl Jung's concept of the conscious mind (the mother), the subconscious (the child) and the superconscious (the father).

The fundamental principle common to all ancient philosophies is that each microscopic part, though unique, comes from the whole and reverts to the whole in time. Therefore each part must be considered in relation to the whole and is a mirror of the whole. Each living part contains within itself the potential for growth, change and death. That is to say, it contains the ultimate yang (creative force, positive force, space, antimatter) and the ultimate yin (death, negative force, density, substance) held in the tension which creates its own unique form.

The more I looked at this principle, the more it reminded me of what I had found to be true during my days making documentaries about social affairs for the BBC. One small element of individual behaviour, replicated in similar circumstances up and down the country, and the reaction to it, rapidly created a political and economic 'phenomenon'. The story of our society is the story of our selves.

So if I applied this principle to my immediate situation, I could say that all the emotional tensions I was witnessing in my family around me in the early days of my illness were in some way replicating me, even though it wasn't easy to see how. If I could step inside and have a look, then perhaps I might find a way to sort out the problems.

One particularly dark and desperate day I was drifting aimlessly through a bookshop when a book cover seemed to leap out at me from the stands.

Without knowing why, other than that it had a pretty cover, I bought a copy of *The Rainbow Healing Journey* by Brenda Davies.

Brenda Davies trained and practised as a psychiatrist but she happened also to be the daughter of a healer. Her mother, in other words, was an expert in perceiving the human energy that has been ignored by orthodox Western medicine and psychology. For many years Brenda kept her knowledge of healing quiet from her colleagues, because the approach is an anathema to the 'scientific' principles of treating mental health with pharmaceuticals to restore the mind's chemical balance. Nevertheless, her clinical experience kept bringing her back to healing.

She found that her knowledge and understanding of the body's energy centres were decisive in unlocking emotional memories, which could be released once they were identified. The most effective tool she used was the Hindu map of the *chakras* in the body and the patient's corresponding experiences, memories and beliefs.

I began to read more about the *chakras*, an ancient concept that has been interpreted in a variety of ways. They embody a level of energy so subtle that there is no instrument to measure them with, other than the human mind and experience. Yet the most powerful part of our experience is immeasurable. Given life, itself unquantifiable, we are then guided and prompted by love, or the absence of it. We know when we have it, just as we feel it when we don't, but no one will ever measure it. So when it came to a map of the variations in our energy, different interpretations didn't bother me. I simply took the ideas that I responded to and tried out the experience.

The beauty of the *chakra* map is the way it mirrors the relationship between forms of energy that we *can* measure and the human body. So just as light splits visibly into the seven colours of the rainbow when it meets 'resistance' that bends it, or sound vibrates at different levels that we divide into seven and call the notes of an octave (the last note in an octave is the same as the first at double the frequency), so these different densities of light and sound are reflected in our bodies. ➤ This is a sequence that we instinctively recognize as harmony, creating peace and balance. This is a sequence that accords with the logical mathematical beauty that is expressed in every part of our world, from the division of cells in biological growth to the spiral sequence of measurements that was detected in natural structures by Fibonacci in the 13th century.

I found the idea that the *chakras* in human beings develop as the child grows especially interesting. If you divide your first 21 years into seven, then the development of each *chakra*, from conception to your maturity covers three years. Your emotional experiences and reactions during each period of three years will have a significant effect on your understanding of the aspects of human existence you are learning about during that time. We grow emotionally like beans on a trellis. The questing tip of the bean is looking for love, for approval, for acceptance, because that is the medium that nourishes us. As we grow through childhood, we shape ourselves around emotional reactions, and we develop kinks the way a bean does, making decisions about how things need to be in order for us to be loved. Later, we forget about those decisions, but they affect every aspect of the experience we were growing through at the time we made them. They affect the way we behave when similar issues recur in our lives, the way people behave towards us, even the people we attract. When we go back to explore our 'kinks' we may discover – as I was about to – that we have been living our adult lives on the basis of the decisions of a three year old. You'll find a summary of the chakras and their associations in the chart on page 223.

Inspired by Brenda Davies' approach, I began to do a kind of 'targeted' meditation. I started with the root *chakra*, at the base of the trunk, which is the *chakra* associated with your formation as an individual, so it relates to your connection with (and separation from) your mother, and everything else to do with your security: your home, your job and money. The root *chakra* develops between conception and the age of two or three. It is the densest part of your energy and so vibrates to the colour red and the note middle C.

I settled myself down, relaxed my body and imagined myself in a completely red world, as though floating in a warm red cloud. Then I searched and brought to mind my earliest memory. The most immediate one was of being bound and gagged in my high chair. I followed my imagination and let myself slip into the mind and body I had then. I was in the dining room of the English cottage we lived in. The table with the remains of a meal was below me and, in spite of the red cloud I had started with, I could clearly see the green distemper wall in front of me. My brothers and a friend, who had been laughing and shouting as they fiddled around my chair and trussed me up, had gone outside to finish their game. They were the cowboys and I was the squaw. It was quiet and the room was empty. I was struggling for breath, urgently trying to shout for my mother, who was in the kitchen next door, but the gag prevented me. I felt the intense panic of being stuffed out of sight and hearing. For a minute or two I was the helpless three year old again, weeping hot, bitter tears. Other times my brothers and this friend had stifled me flashed through my mind. I remembered being trapped under a mattress they were all sitting on, feeling they were squeezing the life out of me. Mine was a voice that my family didn't want to hear. I recognized how often they tried to silence me and how brutal this experience felt.

In this meditation, I was an emotional child, but I was also my adult self, looking at these events from a distance. My mind was moving so fast that I was able to look on this children's game with understanding for the boys whose victim I happened to be. I could fly over the scene and jump into their minds and hearts. Now, I could mentally scream my indignation and hurt at the things they had done, but then ask them why they had behaved this way and listen quietly for the answer. I was surprised at first to hear how quickly and clearly the answer came. I understood how each of them had his own sense of loss and pain, loss of the family in Burma, loss of my father, loss of the warmth of south-east

Asia. For them this change in circumstances coincided roughly with my birth. I could see that their hostility wasn't personal. I was just the smallest available target for their frustration and anger. And I could see how I invited this treatment, because I wanted so much to be loved and accepted as part of the family that I allowed them to treat me this way. And I saw how consistently, in my adult life, I had been demanding the right to speak, while believing I wouldn't be heard. I needed instead, I could see, to explore my version of truth freely, and trust that ultimately it would sound a note that was welcome.

Once I had understood, I was able to let this image of my brothers go, imagining them like helium balloons drifting away in the sky. I cut the ties that bound me to them and came to myself again, opening my eyes and feeling secure in my place on the earth. I had brought up a moment of fear and anger and now that I had felt its fresh bitterness, it was gone, released into the past, with no power to stir me any longer. I felt something melt when I thought of my brothers. Some tiny hard layer of my being dissolved in compassion and love for them that I had never felt before.

This little memory opened the door to many more. I was astonished at the intensity of the feelings that bubbled up when I revisited memories in this way. For a few minutes they were as raw as the moment they occurred, but I would always enter the mind of the person who had hurt me. And it would be as though we were able to say all that had not been said at the time. I was able to feel my pain, understand their pain and, crucially, understand the reaction that I had been carrying with me ever since. When there was nothing more to be said, and I transformed this person into a big helium balloon, cut the tie that connected us, and watched them float away, I was letting go of my old understanding too, leaving room for something new. I could choose to change my mind and live my life in a different way. I was left feeling secure, calm and content, like a shipwrecked survivor on dry land.

I came to call this targeted meditation my 'old wounds' meditation. I recommend this process to anyone who is going through any physical or emotional difficulty. It is the quickest, most direct way to see who you are, to recognize some of the 'kinks' you've picked up that have formed your way of looking at the world, and to *release* them. In the process of releasing them you free not only yourself, to take a different point of view that might suit you better, but you also free the other person in your memory who was trapped in the position of mirroring your expectation of them.

I went on with this process for many weeks, sitting alone in my room, working through different experiences and ages, apparently going nowhere but travelling through decades and continents in my mind. I focused on one *chakra* until I felt it was exhausted before moving on to the next one. It felt so satisfying, like unravelling a knot from the inside, and I was perpetually astonished by how much the opportunity to step into someone else's shoes and see a situation from their point of view was showing me about myself. It was like looking at the tendrils of the roots that had formed me. Was it as a child, for instance, that I had learned to distrust my imagination?

I remembered, vividly, playing with one of my brothers in the back garden of our house, aged about five. We were running around inventing situations that made the drama of our play, calling out to each other the new ideas we had, or so I thought. But then suddenly he turned around, with a vicious frown on his face, and spat at me, 'Stop saying "Let's pretend"! If you say that one more time, I'll never play with you again.' Ironically this brother has spent his life in a land of his dreams as a poet and a painter. Clearly my offence as his playmate was to attempt to interfere with *his* imagination, but as a child I understood that it was better to keep my imagination under wraps.

I knew I was travelling in my imagination now, but I was revelling in it. It was as though I was allowing myself these imaginary legs for the first time. It struck me how foreign this experience was to my education and environment. Everything I had ever been taught put analysis and logical thought at the summit of human ability. Imagination was associated with children and girls, who did not have so much to offer in the society that I grew up in. A girl who wanted to make herself the equal of boys, as I longed to be the equal of my older brothers, would do well to keep her imagination out of sight, or so I understood. Yet now I saw logic as the protector, the part of the human mind designed to keep us safe. Important, of course, but dead, without imagination. Imagination is the creative force in us. I could feel the power of it filling my mind. I grew bolder to let myself travel further with this indefinable power and found an even greater surprise in store.

I allowed myself to use my imagination to go deep into the earliest link with my mother that I had no conscious memory of. I hesitated at first, but then I gave myself permission to continue, reminding myself that I wouldn't be using this information to testify in a court of law, only to explore and see if there was some way in which I could understand her better.

I knew that my mother's marriage was over for her emotionally by the time I was born. When my eldest daughter was born, my mother came to my bedside in hospital and told me how my birth had been for her.

'You were late. Very late. You were ten months in the womb. And then when you did come, the labour was so long and I was on my own. Your father had gone on. He couldn't wait for you to arrive.'

I was born in the Kandang Kerbau Hospital in Singapore. My father was transferred to Indonesia from Burma and the medical facilities in Singapore were deemed to be the best in the region. So my mother left Burma and travelled with my brothers and our Burmese nanny to Singapore to give birth to me before going on to join him in Indonesia. No doubt she felt unsettled and isolated giving birth there, far away from all her family. These feelings were replicated exactly in the circumstances of my birth that she remembered: 'They put me in the room where the fridge was kept, and I just lay there for hours and hours while the nurses and doctors kept coming in and out to get things out of the fridge.' Good facilities. No human contact.

'And you took *so* long to come. They put my feet up in stirrups and they tried to induce you, but I was still in labour for 24 hours!'

I returned to this scene in my meditations and I felt my mother's desperation and loneliness at the time of my birth. I sensed the desire in me to protect and take care of her, and as I did so I realized how this decision had been reflected in our lives ever since, to the point that I was now the only one of her children who lived close to her, or even in the same country. I could see that circumstances that I had recently felt to be a burden on me and a source of resentment were in fact the result of choices that I had made. It was open to me to make a different choice if I wished to, but it was not my mother's fault that I had made the choices I had. It was simply that my freedom of choice had been invisible to me because it was made so far back in the history of my consciousness I could no longer see it. I was beginning to discover the maturity of the infant human spirit and with it the complexity of human life.

Several years after this experience, I found that the relationship between my mother and me is reflected in astrology. My natal chart shows my mother's birth sign, Cancer, sitting on my mid-heaven, which my astrologer interpreted as meaning that I chose, by the timing of my birth, to carry my mother on my back. This gave me a glimpse into the monumental implications of the belief that the energy of the stars is within each of us and reflects choices that we made before birth. Here is one way in which your focus on the microcosm within you, on, for example, your individual emotion at the time of your birth, delivered back to your consciousness by your imagination, can lead you to jaw-dropping vistas of the macrocosm you inhabit. Your life is truly the reflection of a miraculous order we are only beginning to appreciate.

At the time of these explorations into my root *chakra* I was simply concerned with resolving and releasing the anger that had grown up between my mother and me. I did as I had done with the memories of my brothers. I talked to her in my imagination. I listened to her worries and her desires and I forgave her for decisions that *I* had made. When I felt there was nothing more to be said, I cut the cord that bound her to me. I watched her float over the horizon and I felt a deep sense of strength and peace.

I continued doing this with my image of my mother because I enjoyed the process of understanding and release. I had no greater expectations, except that I was happy to be able to let go of the hurt and anger that had grown up between us. In doing so I could look at the choices I'd made and resolve to make some different ones. Opting for what I really wanted would mean there would be no anger in the future and that would suit us *both* better. My mother knew nothing about what I was doing, and I wouldn't have dreamed of telling her. Although I felt no bitterness towards her, we didn't have a level of trust where I felt she could listen to my point of view or try to understand me. I was fighting for my health and happiness and this was a job I had to do for myself.

One day, however, the phone rang, just after I had finished my morning meditation. It was my mother, calling from Spain, where she had been for a few weeks.

'I just wanted to say I'm really sorry for the way I've treated you in the past.'

I was shocked. My mother is a fighter. She's never been known to be ready with apologies. In fact, I don't think she had ever apologized to me before. Conflict just makes her fight harder. But I felt the sweet relief of this kindness flood over me.

'Thank you.'

I felt light like a feather. I couldn't believe this change in tone from her but I knew, also, that it was not an accident. Silently, and privately, I had been releasing the emotional ties that had kept us struggling in a tug of war. When I dropped my end of the rope there was no battle to be had. It astonished me that the energy that this released had somehow become apparent to my mother, whether she was conscious of it or not. Nonetheless, it produced a result that was beyond anything I expected.

'So this stuff really works,' I said to myself as I put down the phone.

This episode began a process of unravelling a knot in this key relationship with my mother that has been profoundly important. It took a little time before I felt able to lower my defences with her, and, just occasionally, I have had to rebuild them. Even so, I have never felt the anger or bitterness I had previously experienced since those journeys through my mind to discover my mother's true nature and understand the pressures upon her which surrounded me as I grew up with her. We have been able to speak frankly to each other of our love and mutual care in a way that had been obscured by years of tension.

When I began to meditate, my mind would often produce a frantic yellow monkey. He would appear almost as soon as I closed my eyes to begin, careering around with crazy antics and jabbering urgent information, as though his life depended on preventing me from exploring anything beyond him. Which, in a sense, it did.

'It's all very well,' the monkey would say, 'but this breathing in and out business is a bit *boring*. I know how to do it without thinking. And I'm more important than that. I have things to do. Essential things. Watch me.' And he'd be off again with a few more comments and plans. I discovered that I could speak to the monkey directly, ask him politely to clear the stage. When I did this he would react with a wounded air. 'But I thought you wanted me there!' Nevertheless, if I insisted quietly, he would slope off into the wings and let me explore the bigger picture behind him.

Once I had been through the process of the 'old wounds' meditation, I found that my body and mind were much quieter. It was easier for me to be still without distraction. The monkey didn't rear his head so often. I realized he had been trying to protect me. He was the logical part of my mind protecting me from feelings I had found painful. When the thoughts and feelings I was uncovering in the different layers of my energy were no threat to me any longer, I didn't need to keep my mind busy to avoid them.

We have a strong inclination to put trouble behind us and get on with life, and of course this is healthy. We learn lessons from conflict and difficulty and they certainly make us stronger. But sometimes we need to review *what* we have learned and see whether the conclusion we reached all those years ago is still useful. We are perfectly free to sweep away the debris, discard old ideas and change our minds.

As I began to change my mind to mirror what I *wanted* to happen, I discovered new consequences. I found myself entering into what I felt was a circle of trust. By allowing myself to experiment, I was unravelling a different experience of 'cause and effect' from the one I had trusted before. It was as though I was taking the blueprint of reality away from the external world of teaching into my own inner authority and changing the results. Yet there were teachers, simply ones deemed unscientific. They spoke of energy and angels, spirits and guides. When I allowed myself to trust their instruction, I arrived at what seemed like a magical outcome.

Driving through Monaco one summer holiday, with our children in the back of the car, my husband was fretting because he couldn't find a parking space. We had driven round the same circuit three or four times and he was by now threatening to turn around and drive home.

That would be a sad end to a day out, I thought, *but no problem. I've just read a book which says you can conjure parking spaces with your mind.*

Silently, I blocked out his seething anxiety and focused all my attention on seeing us glide into a convenient parking space right by the port. Two minutes later, we did.

Results like this were pleasing, even if there was still a possibility that they were entirely random. I was beginning to get a hint of the power of each person's mind to influence events around them and this was too exciting to be wasted very often on parking spaces. Mentally, I felt calmer and clearer. Physically, I still had severe problems to overcome. My desperation to find a way out of my physical problems was leading me to trust what I had previously distrusted. This was leading to new experience, when things I had imagined became tangible in front of me, and that was leading to knowledge I could rely on and expect the results to be repeated. All of this was adding up a word I had never previously understood. I could feel the first stirrings of faith.

CHAPTER SIX

Healing: Coming up to Grass

True healing takes place between feeling and thinking.

Kumu Harry Uhane Jim

'Coming up to grass' is the expression Cornish tin miners used at the end of a day's shift when they emerged from the dark narrow shafts hundreds of feet below ground. As they climbed the tunnel towards their homes on the surface, they could smell the grass on the air long before they could see the light.

So it was with my attempt to find a way out of the long dark tunnel that engulfed me. I was prepared to try anything in my search for a way out and I sensed possibilities long before I understood them. I went to many different practitioners for help with the confusing fog of dizziness and pain and exhaustion that had become a regular feature of my life.

In South Africa I saw a *sangoma*, who asked me to 'blow on the bones' which he scattered on the earth floor of his round *boma*, the grass thatched hut of the traditional African medicine man. He said the tumour was slow growing and caused by a blow to my head as a child – I could think of many! This childhood injury was causing me to twist my head. He thought herbs would cure it. I had a deep reflexology treatment in the Drakensberg Mountains that seemed to send me floating over the clouds. I was given Brandon Bays' book, *The Journey*, to read, and became fascinated by the idea of feelings buried in the physical body.

I saw a cranial osteopath, who seemed barely to touch me but successfully released agonizing tension in my neck and shoulders for several days before it came creeping back again. I had acupuncture, which boosted my energy after initially sending it plunging through the floor. I took a course of Chinese herbs that didn't appear to make any appreciable difference. I went to a private doctor for exhaustive blood tests, which showed that I had the vitamin-B levels of a chronic alcoholic – though I scarcely drink. So I took supplements of vitamin B, zinc and evening primrose oil, which seemed to balance out the good and bad days.

Offers of help were fluttering in – in forms that I didn't anticipate much from, but whose effects continually surprised me. I was sincerely grateful for the offers being made so I was happy to try anything to see what happened.

My first introduction to healing in England was through two venerable Victorian institutions. Both were founded in the 19th century by a generation fascinated with psychic phenomena. Their era was the century of exploration into the energy beyond matter, from the theory that all matter consisted of molecules containing atoms, propounded in 1803 by Dalton, to the generation of an electric arc achieved by Davy in 1810. By the middle of the century, discoveries of the energy *between* tangible substances were being put to practical use. The effect of light on silver nitrate was being used by Daguerre to develop photographs in 1838, and electric arc lighting was used by the Paris Opera House in 1848.

So many practical and revolutionary techniques stimulated that generation's fascination with the power of the unseen. In Britain, it was an age of almost universal belief in God, the Holy Spirit and angels, so that the notion of being able to communicate with these bodies in space was not strange, although it was considered taboo unless it happened through the medium of the established Church.

The Spiritualist Association of Great Britain began life in 1872 as the Marylebone Spiritualist Association, devoted to exploration and communication with spirits in the afterlife. The fact that they have managed to survive to this day, in spite of all the social changes that have swept around them, suggests an enduring fascination with this type of communication. It is a part of human experience that is still taboo as far as discussion in public media is concerned, but it sparks undying curiosity in those who have been touched by it. One of these, considered the benevolent godfather of spiritualist or psychic associations in Britain, because of the large sums he donated to them, was the creator of Sherlock Holmes, Sir Arthur Conan Doyle.

Perhaps it was the white marble bust of him, nestled among the red velvet curtains of the reception rooms in 33 Belgrave Square, that gave the Association the reassuring feel of a nostalgic relic of Edwardian London. I had been introduced to the Spiritualist Association by my half-sister, who was on a quest to connect with the important people in her life. Her mother died very suddenly when she was five and she had little or no recollection of her. Now in her thirties, she was suffering a crisis and needed some guidance to explore that connection. Benevolently overlooked by the oil portraits of famous psychics that gazed from the walls, we joined a queue and trooped into the hall to watch a medium demonstrate her art.

The Association offers daily open demonstrations of mediumship with the intention of showing: 'evidence to the bereaved that man survives the change called death and, because he is a spiritual being, retains the faculties of individuality, personality and intelligence, and can willingly return to those left on earth, ties of love and friendship being the motivating force.'

The 'performance' of mediumship on stage seems like another relic from the days of music hall, and we lurked at the back, wondering if the blonde lady medium would focus on us and illuminate anything for my sister. She hovered and swooped over the audience, sometimes seeming to cast out names or domestic details like bait, waiting for someone to rise and take them. I was sceptical. It was hard to see how her focus could be sharp enough with so many people in the hall for anyone to receive anything useful. It was entertaining to watch in the spirit of the funfair, but so veiled in vague possibilities that it came across like a carefully contrived magic trick.

Yet though the activities of the Spiritualist Association didn't seem quite to cut it for my sister or me, this was the place where I had my first experience of healing. The Spiritualist Association also offers: 'spiritual healing to those suffering from dis-ease, whether in mind, body or spirit, in a warm and loving environment.'

Before we left, I went down to the basement and waited my turn to disappear behind a curtained screen with a volunteer healer. When the moment came, I sat on a chair in the cubicle and quickly whispered my problem.

'I've got a tumour, in my brain, deep inside next to the pituitary, and it's pressing on the right optic nerve.'

It felt strange imparting this information to someone I'd never met before and asking for her help. I was habitually self-contained, not often sharing my feelings with my family – let alone strangers. I was beginning to prise open the doors. My healer looked a bit nervous as she asked me to sit back in the chair and close my eyes. But as she put her hands over my head, I felt a soothing wave of something like light and power stream into me. I was surprised by how comforting the experience was and I tried to remind myself of the feeling afterwards, encouraging myself to think of it as something that had dislodged the tumour and was starting to get it moving out of the way.

I carried on with my attempts to seek some orthodox medical treatment for my condition. But healing had got my attention. My recognition and understanding of the power of healing felt dramatic, but it came at the end of a long process of exploration, not at the beginning. My healers all nudged me towards this understanding, and the process was a bit like the discovery of Andrew Wiles' 'room'. I was just becoming dimly aware of the furniture.

In spite of all these treatments, my health steadily deteriorated until I was depressed and occasionally despairing. I often felt as though someone had pulled a plug out and all my emotional and physical energy had drained through the floor. Meanwhile the hospital scans, when I *did* get to see the results, showed that the tumour was steadily growing. Gloomily, I tried to calculate my future. I took my troubles to my GP and he prescribed anti-depressants. Instinctively, I felt this would make things worse and I decided not to take them.

A year after the diagnosis, I went off in desperation to another venerable Victorian institution in London that my sister had introduced me to. Housed in a comfortable 19th-century terraced house in the shadow of the Natural History Museum, the College of Psychic Studies is a conventional-looking door that opens onto a wild world of possibility. Its founders, in 1884, had a scientific curiosity to explore communication beyond the known physical limits of time and space and the laws of matter. Today the college is mostly devoted to healing and clairvoyance but it holds lectures by a dizzying variety of teachers who offer their personal perspectives on human experience, as well as courses teaching spiritual healing.

I presented myself as a candidate for healing by one of the students. I whispered what I wished to have healed to her in a crowded darkened room where our chairs were isolated only by the now-familiar hospital screens. As soon as she held her hands over me I felt tears well up and roll down my face until my nose and eyes were a running stream. Heavy black clouds seemed to press on me and it felt at one point as though there was an external pressure that threatened to choke me. When my healer held her hands above me and asked for help for me it felt as though I was being taken to a protective space where all I could do was howl like a baby. It was a depressing experience and yet I recognized at once that this could be the help I needed. I realized how isolated I had been feeling, in spite of my family.

This dark experience stirred feelings at my core that I needed to pay attention to. That night I dreamed I was trying to vacuum fallen leaves in the street, but as fast as I cleared them away, there were more leaves falling. I was aware that I would never be able to clean the street and that meanwhile there were tubs of bamboo that needed my attention. This bamboo had been lush and flourishing, but I had let the roots go dry and the plants were nearly dead. I understood in the morning that I had been concentrating my effort on externals which flow continuously in a cycle that was too powerful for me and I needed to pay attention to the root of the matter. I saw that the dream was telling me that forgotten things were important and needed to be remembered to put things in order. I also found that I was feeling better.

I made a decision that I recorded in my diary: 'For the record, 20 November 2003 is the day that I turned around and faced the tiger that is the lump inside my head – and I have an angry elephant in my belly to meet it with.'

A week later I wrote: 'I don't think we're going to be able to do much about my tumour on the physical plane, so I need to tackle it on the spiritual plane.'

Nevertheless, the world seemed fuzzy, although in flashes of clarity I knew exactly what to do. My intuition was speaking to me and I could hear it, but I was unfamiliar with its voice and I scarcely recognized it, so I was quick to doubt it. In addition, the physical and emotional states I experienced were intensely painful. It felt as though I was going through the full cycle of a psychic washing machine. I understood more and more of my buried feelings, but it felt like I was in a bleak place.

However, my dreams had begun to change. Instead of nightmares, I was now discovering an inspiring inner world of light. One night I saw a vision of the sweet angelic face of a little girl whose light was sparkling from her eyes like fireworks. When I awoke I perceived this vision as guidance that the purity and clarity of that bright innocence would get me through this experience of illness and that I would be fine – alive, not threatened, and neither brain-damaged nor disabled. So it has proved to be.

It wasn't easy for me to find this innocence in myself. Innocence was the equivalent of weakness in my world – either the weakness of being the youngest, or a girl, or of not having enough knowledge. I prided myself on my pragmatism, my practicality. Yet now my practical efforts to conquer my symptoms had come to nothing and I felt as though all the wheels had come off my wagon, in spite of my best efforts. Everything I valued seemed to be breaking apart. I had no job and it was unclear whether I would go back to it even if I was well. I was still writing my book, but writing, reading and researching was a painful process when I could barely see, and when my publisher read my first draft she told me with an ominously pitying look in her eye that my book needed 'work'. I loved this project, but clearly I had some way to go to make it shine for others.

Inside, however, I was discovering a source of hope and strength that seemed to be guiding me forward. Clearly that was something that other people could stimulate in me, through healing. This meant that with their help I was in contact with a force much greater than any I had considered possible before. It was as though I was becoming sensitive to the living breath of this greater force within me, which I could choose to call God, or the Divine, or anything else I wanted, but my experience of living was being transformed. No one was more surprised than me.

They say that African *sangomas*, rudely called 'witch doctors' by Christian missionaries working in Africa, begin their training in healing and the use of herbs when they are called to the profession by illness. Usually this illness takes the form of some injury to the head. Gradually I was becoming aware that the tumour in my head was not an annoying irritant that I would need to bypass to survive, but was indeed the heart of my survival. It was a confused picture, but new realizations began to come thick and fast.

One of them was that I needed to ask for help – not just from conventional medical sources, but from everywhere, in any direction. So I began to pray to this mysterious force that I dimly perceived might 'know' more about my life than I did. I prayed to whatever it was that gave me answers in dreams or moments of inspiration as to the way forward. It seemed that when I asked directly in spoken language for what I wanted, I would get it, even if I was apparently talking to the ether. I sensed in the response the feeling of not being alone and I felt that I glimpsed for the first time ever what the Biblical essence called the Holy Spirit was. And as I opened myself up to help, healers suddenly manifested around me from everywhere.

A few weeks later, at a Buddhist centre in London I met Lho Khanseng, a Tibetan medicine master, who had just arrived from Tibet. He was there to offer the empowerment of the Medicine Buddha, considered a most profound blessing in Tibetan Buddhism. To the sound of trumpets and a ceaseless flow of verbal images, simultaneously translated from Tibetan to English, Lho Khanseng presented a picture of the Medicine Buddha to his audience. Lho Khanseng is a thickset, swarthy man, with a thin handlebar moustache and sunburned skin, but he told us to see in him the slim, sky blue Buddha, dressed as a simple monk and holding a bowl full of nectar with infinite power to heal. The chanting continued ceaselessly while we filed up in turn and bowed in front of Lho Khanseng as he touched each one of us on the forehead with a ceremonial vessel, and it was easy to see this image of the Medicine Buddha in him. Afterwards he told us to hold the details in our minds, so that if we closed our eyes we could see the sky raining this image upon us.

'Imagine', he said, 'the Buddha whose body is blue and who sends blue light from his heart to yours, floating towards you so that the light of your hearts mingles and becomes one, like snow falling on an ocean.'

I found the beauty of this melting image so powerful that for days afterwards I scarcely needed to sleep. When I awoke early in the morning and closed my eyes to begin my meditation, I saw a light inside so bright that I was surprised to find it was still dark when I opened my eyes. Over the following months, I held this image to me as a consolation when I felt despair or pain closing in, and although the brightness dimmed a little, the sensation of compassion and optimism was always in me when I captured the image of the Medicine Buddha in my mind.

I still wasn't looking for healing but it presented itself in unexpected ways. Sometimes the experience was uncomfortable. One dark December evening I met my sister for a treatment she had arranged for me as a Christmas treat. I had spent the day in the library tracking down some final bits of research. It's difficult to overstate how depressing some days of research can be. You go through the process of ordering up the books and documents you need – far too many for you to do anything more than skim them frantically in a race against the clock before the library closes and you have to factor another day into your plans. You read intensely, urgently, hunting for the links you need, feeling despair when you fail, willing yourself not to be diverted by a far more entertaining story that you come across, or curiosity about your neighbour's nostril hair. You take detailed notes of tangential matters because, if you don't, you can be sure that these will be the references you need when you think the day's work over at leisure. And, in my case, you debate all the time whether it is better to see one thing at a time but not very much, with a patch on your nose, or see everything at once in a dizzying array, as your eyes try to focus in two directions. By the time I met my sister at the end of the day I was looking forward to a nice relaxing massage where I could lose myself in sensuality.

I hadn't reckoned with Natalia. I had never met anyone quite like her. She welcomed me into a comfortably furnished front room in West London, complete with toning brown leather sofas, conch shells and creamy ostrich eggs. The only incongruous element was the massage couch in the middle of the room, though hardly surprising since this wasn't in fact Natalia's home but a flat she borrowed once a month for a week of back-to-back treatments. I was surprised not to be asked to take off my clothes and instead to lie barefoot on the couch. Natalia covered me up with blankets and I closed my eyes, settling back for a long soothing session.

'Ha!' said Natalia, as she grabbed my right foot. 'There's real conflict here. Teuch! It's deep. It goes back a long way. A long history of conflict with men!'

I never thought I was in conflict with them. I always thought they were in conflict with me! I was thoroughly on edge as Natalia proceeded from my right foot to my left.

'Your spirit is fundamentally compassionate and soft, but it's overlaid with this conflict, which is something you've imposed on yourself since about four years old. It's blocking your creativity which needs to get out.'

Still with my foot, Natalia began to reach 'inside', in some way I could feel but not fathom.

'There's so much sadness in your foot. Exhaustion.'

As she spoke, the room filled with dark grey shadows. Natalia moved up to my chest and began to press rhythmically on my breastbone, leaning over my head and moving up and down as though she was kneading dough. She stroked up from my breast around my neck. It was a strange sensation, breathless but almost comforting, like drowning in the rushing sea. Then she began to pull stuff out of my chest like oversize clumps of wool – stinking strands of dirty laundry.

'You have a lot of anger in you. Anger at your husband and his work.'

'He doesn't work.'

'He doesn't want to, or he can't?'

'He has a lot of pain from his back.'

'Back pain is associated with feeling superior to what you're doing.'

My husband is an intelligent, creative man who had a Saturday job selling light bulbs in an electrical shop.

'A very intelligent person who's doing less than he's worthy of,' Natalia went on, without me speaking. 'Still, you've accepted your situation and realize nothing will change him, short of a miracle. But it's very grey in there,' pointing to my stomach.

I was feeling pretty bad by this time, even worse than when I went in, so I explained about the tumour in my head and asked her what she thought I should do.

There was silence. Eventually, she said, 'There's nothing much you can do except follow the path you're on and find your own way.'

When the treatment was over I felt two inches tall. Was I really in such a dark place that I could fill a room with my sadness? I heard my sister and Natalia exchanging laughter when she went in for her treatment. How much more pleasant it must be to work with my beautiful sister than to have to wrestle with all the grey muck she found in my stomach. What was all this about anyway? How did she seem to know so much about me when I knew so little, and how could I follow the path I was on when I had no idea what it was?

It consoled me a little when my sister came out and told me Natalia said I was a light being, someone who radiates light around them. I didn't understand what that was, or how I could be when the view from inside was so dark and confusing, but I had seen enough of Natalia to realize she knew what she was talking about. And when we went out for dinner I found my right eye was miraculously focused!

When I left Natalia I was feeling like a bedraggled remnant in a psychic laundry basket, but over the next few days I could feel buried clouds lifting from me. I was deeply impressed by the accuracy of her perception of my emotional make-up, presenting me with a picture I had never been able to see myself. The way I had come to see the world had seemed like the only reality to me. My encounter with the power of the intangible energy of healing through her wisdom and perception and the mysterious power of the Tibetan Medicine Buddha left me feeling hugely optimistic for the first time since the tumour was diagnosed nearly 18 months earlier.

Healing, which had been such an unlikely mystery to me, now seemed to be all around. My sister-in-law had studied *reiki*. I knew so little about it that I thought it was a form of massage – but I accepted when she offered me a treatment over Christmas. She burnt sage to cleanse the room we worked in before she began and explained that she would use Sanskrit symbols as she worked to focus the healing energy. It sounded impossible to me that the position you held your hands in could have a significant effect on the healing energy. I wanted to ask, why do you think it works, how does it work and how do you know? But then I had to admit that the healing I had experienced so far had had effects that reached far beyond my understanding of what was possible. I looked at my sister-in-law and saw how the intention to heal lit up her whole being, so that she seemed to grow beyond the personality I had known. So I just closed my eyes and let myself float into the music that was playing in the room.

I had a strange sensation of floating. When she put her hands on my hips the feeling became intense, as though I was floating in the womb, surrounded by amniotic fluid. I felt curiously lost and abandoned, as though stranded at birth. Was I drifting back to feelings I had had at that time or was this just a reflection of my current state of mind? That empty sensation stayed with me after we closed the healing session, and although I was relaxed, I was also sure that I didn't like it.

A little while later a neighbour came to lunch and we talked about healing. Barry said he'd been told he had a facility for it and put his hand over the back of my head. The warmth from his hand seeped under my skull and the nerves in the back of my neck seemed to unfurl and respond. Soon after he left, however, I felt so exhausted and dizzy that it seemed my body wanted to turn inside out. A headache sprang up and lurked with varying degrees of intensity for several days.

Now I began to wonder if healing could be dangerous. I plunged from elation to despair with alarming speed and, curious though I was about the way in which strangers could affect the condition of my mind and body, I feared it also. People seemed to have the power to make changes but not to explain them. Of course I wanted to be in a safe world that conformed to the one I had always known. Could healing make the spirit more open and vulnerable but leave it directionless and exposed? Even so, there was a small voice of optimism that had spoken inside me and its tone was as clear as a bell: *I think I will get better*, it said, *but I feel it's going to be a painful process.*

I had embarked on a path I was hungry to know more about, and I began to pursue it with energy that became more focused as the medical system seemed to descend into chaos around me.

Only a few days later I met a local healer who my friends had recommended to me. Julie was a matronly looking blonde who wouldn't have seemed out of place at a meeting of the village bridge club, but she said that she came from a long line of clairvoyants and healers. In our preliminary conversation she was remarkably quick to pinpoint things that had been on my mind that morning.

A key question for me was whether I would go back to work if I got better. I had realized that I was wedded to my job because I felt my family needed the income, but I had come to see that this was not the only solution to my family's need for security. My old habit of trying to calculate the future had become almost obsessional in this uncertain time. I would spend hours making little estimates and scribbling sums on the back of envelopes for one scenario or the other, for plans I would write out and set for myself. The problem was that my plans did not, and never could, include the unexpected. And the unexpected was what I was living through, a fact that I should have become used to but which continued to surprise me at every turn. The more ardently I planned, the less I seemed to have a grip on reality. Of course the reverse was also true. The fainter my grip on security, the more ardently I planned. But as the intensity of my symptoms deepened I began to see that life could not go on as before. If I had, say, 10 or 15 years left, I decided I wouldn't spend any more of my precious life at the BBC.

I was becoming familiar with the different zones of energy in my body, as I was gradually working through the *chakras* in my meditations, but this was the first time I had worked with a healer who approached my body in that way. As I sat on her chair and closed my eyes, allowing her to send energy through the different parts of me, I was able to perceive the echo of what she was doing. I could sense her passage through the root *chakra* and see a bright red glow, and I felt comfortable as she worked through all the *chakras* until we got up to the brow. This *chakra* has the vibration and colour of indigo, but I couldn't see it at all. It felt blocked, as though I couldn't even allow her hands to pass through me there. She moved on up to the crown *chakra*, at the top of the head, but the show was over as far as I was concerned. That was it.

Julie said that my crossed eyes related to something that I didn't want to see in front of me. She took this to mean my relationship with my husband. He was sitting outside in the car waiting for me, fuming after an hour and a half of my total immersion in a world that he saw as full of charlatans, while Julie's husband fluttered about, pleasantly taking care of the 'business' side of things. I wasn't aware that there was something I didn't want to see about my relationship with my husband. I thought I knew our differences and the problems they had caused us intimately. As far as I was aware I just wanted to survive. But it's very hard to judge whether something is there or not when you've been told you don't want to see it. The process of change, even change from illness to health, can feel deeply threatening.

My husband expressed the view that healing is 16th-century witchcraft. He has absolute faith in his

GP, in whatever this doctor tells him to do and nothing else. I would not have been inclined to disagree with that perhaps, in spite of my critical questioning of pharmaceutical companies in the past, but for the fact that all my efforts to find a medical solution to the problems in my body resulted in 'unprecedented' confusion. The people involved were well meaning; they intended to help me and were, no doubt, good at their job, but a combination of accidents created confusion around things that they held to be certain. No verdict could be given on the developments in my head, in spite of the highly sophisticated magnetic resonance images, if the previous sets of scans were lost somewhere in the bowels of the hospital's archive.

So my husband was not best pleased when I sat up in bed one morning and said that I'd decided to go and see a man who would illuminate healing for me like no one I had encountered before. American healer Martin Brofman opened the door to my capacity for healing. He believes that everyone can be a healer and 'anything can be healed'. That is the title of the book that made him famous, based on his experience of healing himself and the healing method he devised.

The Hawaiians say that 'healing happens between thinking and feeling.' My experience with healing so far had led me to many strange sensations, and unfamiliar feelings, but I needed to understand what was happening, to relate it to what I already knew. I was more inclined to trust thinking than feeling. Martin was the person who bridged that gap for me, and made it possible to relate healing to my feelings and to what I already knew about the way my body worked. There is a logical side to Martin's method, and then an aspect that moves way beyond logic. Over 35 years of using and teaching this system, the magical effects of healing have continued to surprise him. When I had got to know him better, I told him about my husband's view of healing.

'No,' said Martin, 'it's not 16th-century witchcraft. It's 21st-century witchcraft!'

Martin's passion for the past three decades has been the study of the power of human consciousness. In the 1970s he was a computer specialist. He worked as a systems analyst for some of the big banks on Wall Street, devising systems that would be proof against hackers by hacking into them himself. That job requires a fine logical mind and persistence in overcoming problems. Martin is blessed with these qualities in abundance and focused them on computer systems until he developed a cancerous tumour on the back of his neck that paralysed him down his left side and grew so much that it threatened to kill him.

He was taken into hospital for an operation to remove the tumour, only to find when he awoke from the anaesthetic that the surgeons had found it inoperable. They told him they could do nothing for him, so that he was to go home and live the few months they expected he had left to him as best he could. They also told him that should he cough or sneeze, he might cut off the blood supply to the brain, which would kill him.

Martin is a funny man and a natural storyteller. My sister had introduced me to his work and taken me along to a couple of his lectures in London. I had laughed at his story about the impact of being told you only have months to live.

'What are you going to do if they tell you that you only have a few months left? How are you going to spend your time? What are you going to eat? Are you going to worry about the nutritional value of your food?

'Of course you're not. You're going to eat exactly what you want. Every meal could be your last one. So I lived on a diet of hamburgers and milkshakes and I was still alive a year later.'

He had promised himself the holiday of a lifetime if he was still alive when the new year came around, so New Year's Day, 1976, found him on a beach on Mauritius. He met a Buddhist monk who was there to teach meditation, and told him of his predicament.

'Cancer begins in the mind,' said the monk, 'and that is where you go to get rid of it.'

So began a long search by a 20th-century American with a daring temperament and a logical mind. The result was that Martin healed himself, the tumour and the paralysis disappeared, his eyesight cleared, and in the process he developed the healing method he calls the Body Mirror System. It is based on the essential understanding of the Hindus and Buddhists of existence as a state of mind. It is consciousness made 'real' by our perception, so that when our perception changes, our reality changes. Martin has mined and distilled the wisdom of this ancient philosophy and translated it into the practical experience of everyday life – so that there are no mystical symbols, no prayers in Sanskrit, no sets of rules and no barriers to any human being who wants to understand. This is an understanding he has sought to convey in the language that is closest to us – the language of our bodies. For me it was something like Buddhism – in English.

I had known about Martin's work for over a year by the time I decided to go and see him for a personal healing. I learned his view of the *chakras*, and I learned, without understanding, about his view that reality as we perceive it is a co-creation where two or more points of consciousness intersect. I liked his direct manner, his wit and his apparent willingness to tackle any question fearlessly. So the question I asked myself was, why had it taken me so long to go and ask him for healing?

Fundamentally it's a matter of trust. Illness of any kind makes you feel vulnerable. You look for someone you can depend on, someone who will take care of you. Our social education has schooled us to trust doctors, but not to trust healers. A diagnosis of a potentially fatal or a permanently debilitating condition induces such fear that you are open to any suggestions from a doctor. In the six months after the diagnosis I would certainly have offered up my head to the surgeon's knife if I had been told that an operation was possible. Again and again I thank my luck for making such a thing impossible. And if I had been willing to sacrifice a part of my body, how could it seem more threatening, to both myself and my husband, for me to open up to working with a powerful healer?

We can willingly allow someone to remove a part of our bodies surgically because we are told it is in our interests, but not to 'interfere with our minds' for fear that we will never be the same again. There is a certain logic in this fundamentally illogical reaction. We know in our hearts that our consciousness is our life. The prospect of someone interfering with our minds seems far more threatening than the prospect of someone removing an arm, or a leg or a breast. Yet this idea is based on an impossibility. It is far simpler to change your mind than to regrow an arm or a leg. If someone influences your thinking in a way that you find damaging, you can change your mind back again. Your consciousness is you and it is all yours, for life. Nothing and no one can take it away from you. There is consciousness in the parts of your body too, but this is something you only see the value of when you don't have it any more.

However, the night before my visit to Martin, I dreamed I had wandered into a shabby charlatan's den where I'd become stuck fast. The impression of needing to 'beware the healer' was buried deep in my unconscious.

The impact that Martin makes on first meeting is disarming: a highly original mind with a highly unoriginal, ribald sense of humour, a generous belly and eyes that dance at a deep level. He made me think of a Middle Eastern carpet salesman, timeless in his wisdom and timeless also in his showmanship. Yet as soon as I sat and talked to him he set about readjusting the state of mind that had made me sick with the practised assurance of a master.

'What can I do for you today?'

I explained about the tumour they had found in my head and the symptoms I was experiencing. He waited until I stumbled into the magic phrase that came uneasily to me: 'I want to be healed.'

'I look upon the body as a point of consciousness,' he explained. 'Tensions within the body are tensions within the consciousness, and the parts of the body where you have disease, or tension, tell a story. A tumour on the pituitary tells a story of not following your passion. You have to focus on what you want for *you*, like the author Tony Robbins says. The resolution of this problem is in your brow *chakra*,' said Martin, 'to do what you want and to do it well and to earn a living out of that. That's what you must do. What was going on in your life at the time of diagnosis?'

I shrugged. Nothing, it seemed to me, or nothing out of the ordinary anyway. Everything was going on as normal. I was just *about* to have time to follow my passion, to fulfil my long-held ambition to write a book, and this diagnosis had been a severe interruption to that.

'It's very important', said Martin, 'to ask yourself what was happening at the time of diagnosis. Your body's symptoms express your unconscious reaction to the circumstances that occur. You can also ask yourself what the effects of the symptoms are and so what the symptoms do for you.'

I nodded, but I was mystified. How could anybody *want* to experience the headaches and the dizziness I had been living with? How could I have wanted double vision and the fear and trauma of a brain tumour? These symptoms certainly prevented me from doing a job I had been longing to move on from, but they also came close to preventing me from doing anything at all, even from following my passion and writing my book! I was English enough to swallow the expression of these feelings and get myself ready for the healing session I had come for.

Martin explained he would hold his hands over the different energy centres of my body, touching me lightly in each place. While he was doing this I would sit in a chair and do nothing, and then afterwards he would discuss with me what he had seen in my energy. This was a strange language to me, in spite of almost six months of reading about *chakras* and a glimmer of understanding of how people could see the body in terms of energy. Nevertheless, when Martin asked me whether I accepted the possibility that I could be healed by him in this session, I said yes. I allowed the possibility, but I think I expected nothing.

When Martin put his hands over me it was like being plugged into a battery charger. I felt an intense electrical current descend through my head, and then I was lost in a space that felt like a tunnel without end. I imagined at one point that I would die in a gutter alone. I felt a deep sense of isolation, with the despair of abandonment rising up in me like dirty water that threatened to engulf me.

When he had finished I heard him whisper, 'You can open your eyes now.' He asked me whether I felt the same or different.

I stood up and walked around the room. What could I say? I felt like Alice in Wonderland. Not entirely marvellous, but my feet seemed a long way away from my body. I was amazed and open, in a way I had not been in our discussions before.

I was even more amazed when Martin began to describe what he had seen in my energy. He rattled through my whole life story.

'Your sense of being nurtured by your mother was a little bit weak. I expanded the energy there, and put your roots deep down into the centre of the earth so that you can feel nurtured and trusting.'

It was true that although I was close to my mother, she hadn't exactly been the nurturing type. In my adulthood I had felt this relationship draining me of energy rather than helping me, but how, I wondered, did he *know*? Was he guessing?

Martin went on to describe other parts of my experience that I recognized, in my everyday life or from a long time ago, until he came to something that started so far back it was almost indistinguishable from my experience of life itself.

'What was your relationship with your father?'

'He and my mother split up when I was very small. I don't remember ever living with him.'

'So were you close?'

'I wanted to be but I never felt I could talk to him. He died six months before these headaches began.'

'You've felt a great sense of separation from your father, and as a result you've had a deep feeling of isolation all your life and a difficult relationship with authority.'

I was choked with an intense sadness as he spoke, even though these facts had been familiar to me all my life. How, I was wondering, could a stranger simply wave his hands over me and see all these childish emotions that were buried so deep that I didn't think they mattered any more? Was I so transparent that I was dragging these feelings around with me? And *did* they matter? Could such ancient feelings really have caused my physical symptoms?

Nevertheless I felt, rather than thought, that whatever I was experiencing was having a profound effect on me. What Martin was saying induced a kind of wonder in me. I felt my habitual control dissolve and an unfamiliar openness steal upon me in his company. By the time he walked me to the door, I was drinking in his words.

'We are all divine. In our culture it is considered insane if you say, "I am God", but in fact it's true. We are all part of God, or the Divine, or whatever you want to call it. So it's true to say, "I am God", just as it's true to say, "You are God".

'Yes,' I said, happily. 'It's a verb. You can conjugate it like any other. I am God. You are God. He, she, it is God, we are God . . .'

CHAPTER SEVEN

More Magic Than Medicine

In the aftermath of my healing with Martin Brofman, I felt as vulnerable as a baby. It was a miserable feeling and yet I knew that something had changed within me. I dreamed I was in a house where the plumbing system was leaking from every joint in the pipework and I found it strange that I had to go up to the attic to fix it. I knew when I awoke that this dream related to the sense I had of old emotions seeping from every muscle, and 'going up to the attic' to solve the problem represented exploring my consciousness. I was astonished, all over again, by the wisdom and eloquence of the images my subconscious mind presented me with when I slept.

When I came to do my meditation in the morning and visualized the centres of my energy, I perceived them as different. The colour of the root *chakra* was a brighter and deeper red and the roots seemed to go deep into the earth. Some colours that I had perceived only indistinctly before now seemed bright and immediate. This surprised me. I could feel a change but I had not expected to 'see' a change in my own energy so effortlessly. It was astonishing to me that this could be the effect of another person using his energy to heal mine.

There was an even greater shock waiting for me when I sat down the next day to get back to work. The first draft of my book about my ancestor, John Parkinson, the herbalist, was finished. The task of revising and editing it lay in front of me and I felt the time to start that had come. I sat down and read the first couple of lines of the preface I had written and stopped. I couldn't believe what I was reading. Or rather, I couldn't believe that I was now understanding what I had written for the first time.

The first page of this book of 180 pages began, 'I never lived with my father.' I had written this because the inspiration for my book about John Parkinson was the 1629 book that was one of my father's most precious possessions. I wanted to explain that it wasn't familiar to me as I grew up because I never lived with him, so discovering the book as an adult had a greater impact on me. Yet now, as I read this line, I saw in it my profound unconscious need to establish links with my father that had never existed for me in his lifetime. I understood that my passion for this book, and the world it connected me to, began after my father died and reflected my deepest feelings that I had failed as his daughter because I had never been able really to communicate with him. That feeling was compounded by the terms of my father's will, revealed six months after his death. He had chosen to leave each of his children different amounts of money. The sums were small and not life-changing for any of us, but it felt to me as though he had just marked my paper. I was back at school and here were the results of the exam I had tried my best to succeed in. Verdict? Better than some, but not the best. B+. Somewhere in middle. The story of my life.

Of course I know that this was not my father's intention. He was merely trying to distribute a small amount of money where he felt there was most need for it, but this didn't prevent me from feeling the pain of what I saw as my failure. I squirrelled the feeling away, ashamed of my childishness, but now I could see that this was the time of the first headache, the earliest symptom of the illness that later manifested as a brain tumour. I could see how my creative work and my illness were all part of the same fabric of a life that had felt profoundly jolted when an unsatisfactory relationship with my father seemed gone forever.

I sat there, digesting the impact of this single half sentence with new clarity. I reflected on some of the curious circumstances that had seemed to lead me on through years of patient sleuthing to deepen my link through my father with this herbalist ancestor and his generation. I remembered the early days of my interest, for instance, when I dropped into a specialist second-hand bookshop in Hay-on-Wye because we happened to be visiting friends nearby. The tiny shop was lined with books of all ages about the natural world, gardeners and natural scientists. Did they, I asked, have any books about John Parkinson?

'No,' the answer came, quick as a flash, 'because there aren't any. But we've got one of his books in the window.'

I had looked into the window, in amazement. John Parkinson wrote two important books in his life, the gardeners' favourite, the *Paradisus*, which was the first book about decorative gardening in English. This had been my father's legacy. And then the book that the apothecary had seen as his life's work, the *Theatrum Botanicum*, his review of the history, characteristics and medicinal uses of more than 3,000 plants, which had taken him over 50 years to complete and which he had finally published in 1640, just before his country collapsed into civil war. Centuries later, a copy of this great book, its original leather binding carefully patched in sections, heavily inscribed with the name of the apothecary who originally owned it, was in my hands being offered to me for sale.

Of course I bought it, and even at the time it felt as though I had somehow been led to it. Looking back now it seemed that this purchase was part of a bigger picture framing my life, which I was just beginning to perceive. I could never understand why no one had written about John Parkinson before, despite generations who had valued his work and even a society founded in his name at beginning of the 20th century. It was a strange feeling that this project, which anyone in the past 350 years could have undertaken, had somehow been waiting for me. Looking again at my manuscript, I felt suddenly connected to something that guided me, whether I knew it or not. I glimpsed a field of energy surrounding my existence on this planet in that moment. Awestruck is probably the right word.

I tried to tell my husband how I felt. He was grumpy. He wanted to be sympathetic to my feelings but the notion of healing made him hostile.

'So do you believe it's worked?'

'What do you mean?'

'It's obvious, isn't it? If the consultant says we have to do such and such, will you say yes or will you say no, I've already been cured?'

'I can't answer that. I don't know.'

'It's a perfectly simple question.'

Lethal logic again. He wanted the situation pinned down. Within minutes we were arguing. I tried to explain.

'This is emotional and psychological work which the tumour has made me do. It's work I'm doing anyway, with my meditation.'

'I know, 'cause you're never there to say goodbye to the children in the morning.'

There were no words to answer. I felt anger and guilt in equal measure. I knew at some deep level that opening up this internal can of worms representing my old emotions was the only way to save my life. It was, after all, the only thing I could do. But not even your nearest and dearest will love you all of the time.

This was a hard lesson for me to learn. I had always wanted to please them, to do the best I could as a wife and mother, to say nothing of the creative work I was employed to do at the BBC. This business of trying too hard was probably what had made me ill in the first place. I had come a long way from making decisions on the basis of what *I* wanted, and I no longer knew what would make me happy. I would not have described myself as a perfectionist, because I was always aware of how far I fell short of that goal. I set myself the grandest goals and then berated myself roundly for failing to reach them.

Later I read a beautiful piece by the writer Annie Lamont in her book, *Bird by Bird*.

> Perfectionism is the voice of the oppressor, the enemy of the people. It will keep you cramped and insane your whole life . . . perfectionism is based on the obsessive belief that if you run carefully enough, hitting each stepping stone just right, you won't have to die. The truth is that you will die anyway, and that a lot of people who aren't even looking at their feet will do a whole lot better than you . . . and have a lot more fun while they're doing it.

I was beginning to focus on the positive things I could achieve with my life and to get the message: enjoy the journey you're on. If you don't like it, change it, and remember: to err is human, to forgive divine. If you're going to unleash the divine within you, you'd better start by forgiving yourself for your mistakes.

I could not answer the question as to whether or not I was healed after my session with Martin. All I knew was that my perceptions of reality were changing profoundly. I felt the vulnerability that comes with being newly made, as though I had just come through the birth canal. My symptoms continued; I felt dizzy and confused. For a while everything in my life was still in pieces.

I had been waiting for the professional view of my most recent scan. When nothing arrived, I rang my consultant's secretary, who I was on first-name terms with by now. For several days she didn't return my messages. Then eventually she contacted me, apologized for the delay, explaining that she'd been on a course, and said my consultant had dictated a letter for me before going on holiday. She would send it in a couple of days, as soon as she had transcribed the tape. A week later I rang again to check on her progress.

'I'm sorry,' she said, 'I don't know what happened. When I got to the end of the tape the letter for you wasn't there. Somehow it didn't record. We'll just have to wait until Mr Powell gets back from his holiday.'

I sighed. This scan had been done a few days after my healing with Martin and I was interested in the results, but once again they had got hopelessly lost. When my consultant returned from holiday he emailed me to apologize for the unprecedented confusion and gave his verdict on my medical condition.

The signs were contradictory, he said, although he couldn't remember the exact details because he had lost the letter he dictated, and, by now, the secretary. He thought this was possibly a rare form of *meningioma* (which is benign), or part *chondrosarcoma* (which is not) and part *meningioma*, or possibly a *haemoangionoma* (which caused the bleeding and the headaches), but in truth they didn't know. At any rate, operating on this area was an unwelcome prospect and they would not advise radiotherapy either in case this tumour was resistant to radio and having it could 'queer the pitch' for surgery later. They couldn't say whether it was growing, although they thought it had grown, and they were too cautious to predict the future.

So, two years after my initial diagnosis, here I was, floundering. I was apparently a lot sicker than when I was first diagnosed. My eyes were completely crossed. I was dizzy on most days. My energy fluctuated violently with devastating drop outs, and the headaches were unpredictably savage. Yet I felt strangely elated.

I could have laughed out loud at the series of misadventures in the medical process. It seemed that I needed all these unprecedented 'mistakes' to finally get the message. I was now wholly convinced that the solution to the problem was within me, and it felt liberating to be able to distance myself from depending on the medical system. I could not blame the hospital for the farcical accidents that kept them from giving me satisfactory answers to the problems I was having. I now understood that these 'accidents' had more to do with me. I was experiencing the truth of what I had often heard: there is no such thing as coincidence.

When something keeps happening to you, it makes sense to ask yourself what you have to do with it. What was there in me that could explain the 'unprecedented' confusion over my symptoms? I had kept trying to give responsibility for my illness to the medical establishment. Events kept on showing me that they could not take responsibility, and landing the problem back in my court. I was lucky, I knew, to have been given so many opportunities to learn this simple message. I was profoundly grateful that surgery had not been seen as the solution to the problem. Yes, I had a brain tumour and my nervous system was not working as well as it was designed to, but at least it was intact. I had seen enough of the after-effects of life-saving brain surgeries on people not to wish it for myself.

In spite of my physical problems, the landscape of my inner world was clearing. I felt as though I knew what I wanted and where I was going. I glimpsed a future in which I was the writer and healer I have become. I wrote in my diary,

> I will tell the pain in people's hearts and also heal it with my hands. What I really want is healing, an end to the pressure, the dizziness, the wonky eyes. I ask Sanjay Menla (the Medicine Buddha) for it and the Holy Spirit. And I am sure that it will happen.

As my inner landscape cleared, my outer world began to mirror it, in small ways at first. I found that I could have a friendly conversation with my mother, after many years of tension. I could see that the book I was writing was a transition between two phases of my life. The earlier half, in which the facts and measures of material reality were paramount, was giving way to another one in which I could see the outlines of a spiritual reality that was more powerful. In this spiritual reality there were different rules. There were no divisions of time and space, for example. It was intangible and seemed like a dream, and yet increasingly my experience was showing me that the world I could touch and move in reflected my state of mind at its deepest level. For the first time I understood what the Buddhists mean when they say that 'Cancer begins in the mind, and that is where you go to get rid of it.' I knew I had work to do.

To overcome the problem, I needed to face the enemy. I realized how much I had avoided thinking about the fact that I had a brain tumour, instead of focusing intently on it. I began to spend ten minutes, three times a day, summoning an image of the tumour, its position and the shivering mass of it. It was like being a very small person standing beneath a mountain of flesh and it was my task to remove it, cell by cell. My mental image quickly turned into a shadowy gardener, digging away at the pile of cells, and trundling them off in his wheelbarrow, naturally – since I was writing a book about a gardener. I began to use every spark of my imagination to help me. If I felt I had a spiritual gardener in my head, able to work on removing the tumour, so what? I had the right to trust my imagination. This decision alone was a novelty for me. I had spent many years in the uncertain landscape of right and wrong. Now I didn't care. I set my gardener to work and tried faithfully to keep my appointment with him, three times a day.

It felt very indulgent, to shut off the world for those regular ten-minute breaks. It seemed selfish, but delicious. A sense of calm and clarity would enfold me as I beavered away at this one simple task. I noticed that life at home worked better, the family temperaments were sweeter, on the days when I kept up this regular regime. Sometimes I would forget, or become so involved in some other task that I didn't break off to meditate, and I began to notice that those were the days when disasters happened. Emerging carelessly from a car park space, I reversed into another car – on a day when I had forgone my regular routine so I could carry on cleaning the car! Shaken up by the accident, I let my evening session go also, for the pleasure of having my daughter throw a hissy fit and march off across the fields in her socks!

I began to notice that my calm and focus created calm and focus around me and my neglect of this simple regime had the opposite effect. That, and a growing confidence that I was making progress, reconciled me to the 'selfishness' of my regular periods of isolation with my meditation.

I was developing a new relationship with my environment. My meditation had led me to understand the deeply personal relationship I have with the earth and the air above me. As a living human being, each one of us is a part of the earth, living out its natural process of creation and death. I watched the birds in my garden sharing this space with me. I noticed their family groups calling to each other from tree to tree; their sense of ownership of their little piece of earth. I saw the way the wrens would occupy one particular laurel bush year after year; the pigeons, the ash tree opposite; the blue tits, the hawthorn in another corner of the garden. I realized these birds and their ancestors had been coming back to the same parts of the garden for longer than we had lived in our house, for longer, even, than the 400-year history of the building. Sometimes I would come out in the morning to find breast feathers strewn across the grass. I felt a personal sense of loss at the brutal end of one of the pigeon family. Those pigeons were like overweight shoppers in a Christmas market, building their comfort apparently with no sense of self-protection. But such a severe end was in itself a message of endurance to me. These birds lived with the prospect of death, overcame it, returned in the spring, adapted their habitat in response to threats or destruction, retuned their call to the new sounds around them, the traffic, the mobile phones, the aeroplanes. While I had no idea whether they felt joy in the process, I knew that seeing them live gave me joy.

My unfamiliar state of openness and sensitivity brought difficulties also. I discovered that there was no difference between emotional pain and physical pain. The relationship became so swift in me that I could not doubt the origin of my pain. As soon as I heard or remembered something that hurt me emotionally, I would feel it in some part of my body, as though I had been punched. Sometimes emotions would well up so intensely that I felt breathlessness choke me. It was like staring into a black chasm, expecting a tsunami to drown me. When these feelings became unbearable, I found a way to use my new understanding of the earth to help.

I would seek out a private corner and stand outside, in my bare feet if possible, reminding myself that while my parents had given me life, as an individual I was a child of the earth. I saw how everything we have comes from the earth, whether it's plants for food or rocks and raw materials for building, or cars. The earth's materials are transformed by human creativity to build an environment that we need, as the birds do. When we have done, our bodies, our cities, and all our creations are absorbed by the earth again, to be reprocessed in time as a source that nourishes, or protects. In this grand perspective, the earth is truly our mother, and I felt gratitude and trust in my place on her.

I allowed myself to talk to the earth out loud, asking for her help. The language I used was my own. It had meaning for me. Then I would close my eyes and mentally travel to the part of my body where I felt pain or tension. When I found it, I would roll the thing up like a piece of old wrapping paper until I had a tight ball. Then I would roll it down through my body and out of one leg, imagining it continuing to travel through the layers of earth, deep into the subsoil below, becoming squashed and distorted in the underground caverns and lakes, beginning to disintegrate in the molten magma, until finally it reached the white hot fire at the earth's core. There, I would see it dissolve and transform into pure energy that feeds and moulds the planet. I imagined this energy like a spear of white fire travelling back up through the layers of earth and vegetation until it reached the sole of my other foot. Then I would watch it travel up my leg and fill my body, going to the place where I had felt the pain. When I was sure it had arrived, I would let out a deep breath and open my eyes.

That was all. The whole process took less than five minutes. The pain would be gone. The feeling would be safely deposited in the earth. As I let the pain and the emotion go, I understood more about why I had felt it in the first place – information that helped me to see how I participated unwittingly in an experience in which I felt like a victim. I came to call this process my 'Earth Healing Meditation'. It worked for me again and again, and when later I began to work with clients as a professional healer, I found it was one of the most effective tools I could give them. It allowed them to strip away layers of pain gradually and safely, as it did me, always providing a safe outlet when something seemed too big a burden to carry.

Gradually, I was beginning to feel physically stronger. My energy was returning and becoming less erratic. I began to listen to my internal conversation. I heard myself say 100 times a day, 'I must do so and so . . .' and I gave myself the chance to change this to 'I want to do . . .' instead, anticipating that the sentence would end differently. But I noticed also my growing inner optimism. Several times a day I would find myself saying, 'I'm so lucky', because my illness had left me with all my limbs intact and at least one functioning eye, and I was convinced I was recovering. My inner musings were even set to music. Jimmy Cliff's version of that old Johnny Nash hit from the seventies rang around in my head:

I can see clearly now. The rain has gone.
It's gonna be a bright, bright, sunshiny day.

CHAPTER EIGHT

Reality, But Not as We Know It

If a man will begin with certainties, he shall end in doubts; but if he will be content to begin with doubts, he shall end in certainties.

Francis Bacon,
The Advancement of Learning, 1605

I was amazed at the transformation in myself and the revelations I was experiencing about how I functioned. I had the sense that there was a part of my brain that had been unused and undiscovered. There was a language just out of my conscious reach that expressed itself in ways I was unfamiliar with. I wondered whether it was music. Sometimes when I woke at night and got up to meditate I heard snatches of symphonies in my head. I slept less and less. I was happy – happier than I had been for years, but I also wondered whether I was going mad.

In the cool light of day I reassured myself that this was discovery, not madness.

'I realize that is the great fear,' I wrote in my diary, 'the chasm that you have to have the courage to go down to reach the mental capacities on the other side.'

To discover the power of your imagination, you have to become like a child again, and proffer your imaginings as truth. The difference between the mad and the mental adventurer is that the adventurers are always aware of the road they have travelled and where they want to go.

Occasionally, there were unfortunate side effects during this time of dazzling exploration. The power of my internal world was so fascinating that I would sometimes forget where I was. Once, I turned a street corner in the car and drove casually into the traffic barrier on the pavement edge before I realized what I was doing. My mind had been distracted by something I had seen on a wall, and I forgot to look in front of me. Although I was behind the wheel, it's true to say there was no one at home! I found it hard to believe that I had done this, but thanked heaven that I hadn't hurt anything other than my car and my pride. After that I made sure to remind myself that my car was like my physical body, a powerful machine that needed my full attention whenever I was using it.

A short time later I found myself working with a group of people who were as comfortable with the language of their imaginations, or intuition, as with any other language they spoke. I was tying up the loose ends of research into John Parkinson, and one of the outstanding things I wanted to find, if possible, was his will. When John Parkinson died, 18 months after

Charles I was executed, there was no government at all in Britain. For two years, until Oliver Cromwell set up his Protectorate, there was no state authority. The king was dead, his court disbanded, the Church abolished and the New Model Army divided. So the wills of people who died during this time, which would normally have gone to the Church court for probate to be proved, ended up scattered far and wide.

I had come across an article by Peter Stewart, a former engineer for British Aerospace, describing the uses of 'remote viewing'. Peter described how he used intuition and dowsing to locate things that were physically beyond view. In 2004 he had organized an experiment to dowse the position and condition of the Beagle 2 spacecraft that was lost on Mars. I wrote and asked him whether he could use remote viewing to find John Parkinson's will. This enquiry resulted in me spending a weekend near Bristol with a group of people interested in developing their remote-viewing skills. On this occasion they would concentrate on remotely viewing the past rather than Peter's more usual territory, which was to help space programmes recover their instruments from distant planets. I took with me the leather-bound copy of John Parkinson's *Theatrum* which I had found in Hay-on-Wye, carrying it wrapped up in a quilt to protect it. I laid it on the table in the room where we met to work, still wrapped, revealing no other information beyond its massive bulk.

One person in the group was an experienced dowser from Devon. She held her hands over the anonymous quilted bundle and said she felt 'a huge information field'. She saw a man in his forties, with short brown hair, and funny glasses, using the book in the back room of an apothecary's shop, surrounded by bottles and jars and 'funny equipment like an alchemist's'. I was impressed, even though I reasoned that she might have heard some of this in advance from Peter. But as the weekend progressed I had to admit that something extraordinary was going on.

Peter's plan for 'remote viewing' was that I should give a place and a date where each person in the group would individually journey back and 'meet' John Parkinson, and then we would all reconvene and share the information we had gleaned from our 'conversations' with him.

I told the group a little about John Parkinson. I had spent more than two years gathering details and I was steeped in information about him, but with this group I restricted myself to the broad outlines of his life: when and where he had lived and what his major achievements had been. We picked May 1630, a year after his first book, the *Paradisus Terrestris*, was published, to meet him in his garden on Long Acre in London's Covent Garden. Then we all shuffled off to close our eyes and transport ourselves into a silent imaginary encounter.

I anticipated this exercise would be a familiar pleasure for me. I had often imagined myself talking to John Parkinson, since the first time I had opened the *Paradisus* to read it. After that, when I walked in my garden or worked with plants that had been his professional and personal passion, I had the sense that he was whispering information in my ear. Even so, I was surprised by what happened when I set out to meet this man on a meditative level.

It was as though I could see and smell the world that he lived in. For the first time, I was visiting *his* world, rather than dragging him into mine. I was able to ask him questions, meet his friends and form a personal impression of them. I revelled in this three-dimensional world I had conjured up, which was feeding me details I had never expected.

I was even more surprised when we reconvened as a group to relate the experiences of our individual encounters with this 17th-century apothecary. I could easily explain the wealth of detail that was apparent to *me* when I met him in my mind, as the result of many months of intensive research during which I had been knitting together the fragments of his life to form a complete story. It was not really surprising that his world seemed so vivid and real to me. Yet when each member of the group began to tell the story of their meeting in turn, I found that each one had turned up some detail about John Parkinson that was unique to him and which they could not possibly have known beforehand.

One woman, for example, had a long discussion with him about different types of manure, a subject in which he was particularly interested since he held great store by the different levels of heat and texture generated in the soil by the manure of different animals. It was a skill he had learned from his horticulturally more-advanced Flemish friends. Another woman was taken to see his rhubarb patch, of which, she said, he was extremely proud. John Parkinson was the first person to grow rhubarb in England, from seeds that were sent to him by a doctor friend who was living in Pisa. Rhubarb was an important medicinal plant in the early 17th century and being able to cultivate a reliable local supply was a significant innovation. There was even comedy in these kaleidoscopic encounters. Only two out of the group of 12 people were men and both of these were greeted by John Parkinson in his formal court clothes, which they were able to describe in detail, whereas every woman in the group described his clothes as a dirty leather jerkin. Evidently the men were important in a way the women were not, so worthy of a special effort!

There was one more journey into the unknown for me before we separated that weekend. We were each to take an object and see if we could mentally tap into its 'information field'. This is the process called 'psychometry', or measuring an object by the mind. The theory is that everything that was ever known or ever will be known exists in some kind of supra-physical space that Pantanjali, the 'father' of yoga, called poetically the 'raincloud of knowable things'. This description of a wondrous treasure trove of information denotes somewhere accessible to each one of us, if we allow our intuition to go there.

I picked up a stick, a solid but ordinary-looking piece of wood, held it in my right hand, the hand I do not use to write with, and closed my eyes. Someone in the room knew all about this stick, but I didn't know who. An image of its owner came into my mind. She was striding uphill through a pine wood on her long legs. I thought perhaps we were in Norway or Sweden. I saw a road stretching uphill in the setting sun. Then I saw a man in green smiling and presenting the stick to the woman after he had used it to draw a circle in the earth. He gave her the stick with love and she felt safe in his love.

I opened my eyes. There was only one woman in the room with long enough legs to be the stick's owner, and it was indeed her stick. It came from a pine wood in Spain, not Scandinavia, and she had gathered it from the hill at El Escorial, where Franco built a monumental cross. She had taken it from under a pine tree and used it as a 'talking stick' so she could talk to the tree. She had asked the tree what she should do and the answer she got was that she had everything she needed right where she was.

I was astonished to find that what had come to me so easily was a mirror of her reality. I had never heard of people talking to trees before then, but it was easy to see that my 'green man' corresponded to her conversation with the tree, and his action in drawing a circle was an indication that she had everything she needed around her. This language of the intuition was new to me and I was only just beginning to discover its power.

I was finding that I could access the power of the mind to travel across physical barriers of time and space, and understanding how this faculty lies within each of us if we choose to acknowledge it. The familiar boundaries of my world were shifting rapidly now that I had encountered this possibility, which I still found astonishing. It was so far removed from my habit of obtaining information through careful research and sources I had checked for 'credibility'. 'Credibility', it now seemed to me, meant someone else's judgement and not my own. I had been more willing to accept the authority of an educational or political establishment than the validity of my own experience.

This glimpse of another way of seeing 'reality' didn't prevent me from seeing things the way I had been trained to by my education. I was still able to make an argument out of provable 'facts' in a respectable academic fashion, and I was careful to do so in the historical biography I was writing. I kept my purely imaginative insights into the subject of my story hidden, like a dirty secret, lest the cultural establishment should greet my book with derision. And yet there was a curious echo between my subject and what was happening for me in my life as I was writing the book.

The purpose of John Parkinson's work, and that of the generation he inspired, was the re-evaluation of knowledge so that it could be of use to his fellow countrymen. He was a pioneer of the scientific renaissance in Britain, exceptional amongst his contemporaries not just for his insatiable thirst for knowledge about plants, but for his insistence on recounting facts learned through direct experience. This was the essence of renaissance thinking that led to a fresh understanding of the world throughout Europe. John Parkinson's generation was one of discovery and innovation, introducing the first bank, the first international trading company, and settling North America. Unfortunately for him, it was also the generation of England's anti-Catholic phobia and civil war. As a result, it was the next generation, that of Isaac Newton and the Royal Society, which laid the foundations of modern science. Yet John Parkinson, a Catholic throughout his life, was an honest observer with a passion for nature who pointed the way to the development of science as we know it in the West.

For hundreds of years in the Western world, 'knowledge' had been considered to be what was written in books. As the few books that existed were written by churchmen, Church doctrine conditioned what could be considered truth. So descriptions of nature were based on belief rather than observation. An animal that had never been seen, such as the Tartary Lamb, a kind of sheep wolf that grew out of the ground like a tree, existed because it was said to exist in a 15th-century manuscript written by an eminent divine. Truth was not so much about 'facts' as beliefs. Sir Francis Bacon, contemporary with John Parkinson and the most eloquent English voice of the revolution in understanding that was taking place, mocked the faults of the formal education system: 'In the universities of Europe they learn nothing but to believe: first to believe that others know that which they know not; and after, themselves know that which they know not' (Francis Bacon, *Filum Labyrithi*, British Library manuscript).

John Parkinson came from farming stock, too poor to participate in 'education', as it was known at Oxford and Cambridge. Even if he had had the resources of a gentleman, his family would have considered such an education useless. People would starve or die of disease if they based their knowledge of nature on anything other than precise observation and experience of animals and plants, and that was not to be found in books, before John Parkinson himself wrote one. Naturally, his work as a herbalist was based on this principle of direct experience, echoing the renaissance that was flowering across Europe.

Now here we were, it seemed to me, coming full circle. We still relied on 'truths' taught at school, over and above direct observation, only now the 'authorities' were no longer divines, but doctors and academics. I read *The Field*, a book in which journalist Lynne McTaggart recounted experiments with an alternative view of physics. To me, a non-scientist, it was a revelation. It seems, contrary to what I was taught, that there is 'something' that exists in a vacuum. Something, called the 'zero point field', is so small and difficult to measure that as a matter of convenience physicists set it aside, a little bit like lopping three noughts off a thousand and calculating in single figures when you mean thousands. Some physicists around the world have considered there might be interesting energetic properties in this zero point field, and although it has been hard to get funding for this research, they have derived promising results in controlled tests from taking into account that what has appeared to be empty space to the most sophisticated instruments we have measured with is not empty at all.

This area of research is not taken seriously. Hence the difficulty in raising funds for it. It made me smile to think of what happened when John Parkinson's contemporary, Dr William Harvey, came up with the novel theory that blood circulates in the body by means of valves along veins and arteries. His fellow doctors warned him he would be considered 'crack-brained' if he published this theory, and that his practice would 'fall off mightily'. He published anyway, in 1628. His practice did fall away, and although for a time he was saved by becoming physician to the king, his theory was not accepted as fact until 65 years after his death. We may be just as slow as our ancestors. What we believe to be true is still a 'belief about truth'. Societies in general are slow to change their beliefs.

Of course, academic doctors and scientists are breaking new ground and making startling discoveries all the time, but it takes a long time to change what we regard as 'true'. Never is this more so than in the way we think of our bodies. Our bodies seem to us quintessentially solid. What could be more reliable, more tangible than your own body? When our bodies break down, we tend to regard the problem as 'out there', not something we own at all. People can become angry with their bodies. Some talk about hating their bodies, as though the mind inside and its physical vehicle were two entirely different things.

Feelings, by contrast, seem fleeting. At the very heights of love or in the depths of despair we are convinced that our view of the world will never change, but then more than ever we can switch from laughter to tears and back again in minutes. Our thoughts come and go. Feelings can be brushed away and buried in physical activity.

The way in which we, and our doctors, for the most part talk about ourselves is couched in a view of biology that conforms to all the old 'laws' of how matter behaves, but it doesn't take into account the new understanding of matter at a microscopic level. All the evidence shows that bodies and feelings are closely interrelated. Our bodies are not as substantial as we imagine and our thoughts and feelings are not so immaterial.

Once my interest in a scientific view of matter had been sparked, physics suddenly became the most fascinating topic I could find. There were 'laws' of physics that I knew about – the very laws of gravity, friction and opposing forces that John Parkinson's generation had begun to determine. Of course we all know these work on the same scale as the one with which we usually perceive the world.

However, there are apparently different laws that govern matter at the microscopic level. At *that* level I was discovering information that distinctly echoed the magical connection I had experienced between my thoughts and the tangible world. The study of matter based on the elementary particles of energy – quantum physics – has revealed a way in which the body, and everything that I had previously considered solid, is as fluid as the mind.

The existence of atoms as the building blocks of matter was suggested long before the dawn of modern science by Indian and Greek philosophers. They take their name from the Greek word *atamos*, which means indivisible. Only, of course, as we all now know, they are divisible. In the late 19th and early 20th centuries, scientists proposed the existence of sub-atomic particles that could, in theory, be separated from the atom. They suggested protons and neutrons in the nucleus of the atom, and electrons suspended around the nucleus. When a machine was developed that could actually see the atom, the scanning tunnelling microscope that was unveiled by two Swiss scientists in Zurich in 1981, it led to the discovery of even smaller parts within protons and neutrons, called quarks.

All these elements of an atom operate in apparently empty 'space' within it. So, even the densest material, where we know the molecules are tightly packed together, contains an empty theatre at its microscopic level that we cannot define. It is infinitesimally small. It takes approximately one million carbon atoms to make up the breadth of a single strand of your hair, and within each atom there is a nucleus, surrounded by electrons moving in 'space', and within each nucleus, there are six neutrons and six protons, surrounded by 'space'. Within the neutrons and protons there are quarks, surrounded by 'space'.

What is interesting is the way the way the building blocks that make up your physical substance, and any substance for that matter, behave at this ultra-microscopic level. They are remarkably hard to pin down. Electrons have an electromagnetic relationship to the nucleus that they respond to, but they can move or join another atom with far less of a pull than that which bonds them to their 'own' nucleus. And they cannot be placed exactly. We know they exist, and their existence makes a material difference to the atom they are bound to, but they are like a wave of energy in perpetual motion. They move around together, held in a wave by an electromagnetic relationship to their nucleus, but the shape of the wave can be changed by photons, which are the smallest particles of light, or another form of electromagnetic radiation. So the act of measurement changes electrons. They exist in a *relationship*, in a 'probable' location. They somehow manage to be matter and energy at the same time.

This is a strange idea to get used to in a world that we have come to understand obeys the classical physical laws of gravity, relative force and so on. All those laws are true, and they work, and yet within all of them, at the very heart of matter, so far as we know, is something that is both matter and energy, and mutable. Even physical matter, with this atomic structure, accounts for only about 4 per cent of the universe as we know it. The rest has no atomic structure. We simply call it 'dark matter'. There is far, far more that we *don't* know about than there is that we do, and what we *do* know about is very hard for our conscious minds to grasp because it seems to contradict every rule by which we function and survive.

This ultramicroscopic behaviour of what is apparently solid was described by one quantum physicist as an:

> utterly bizarre world where nothing is certain and objects don't have physical properties until you measure them. It's a world where distant objects are connected in strange ways, where there are entire universes with different histories right next to our own, and where 'virtual particles' pop in and out of existence in otherwise empty space. (Chad Orzel, *How to Teach Quantum Physics to your Dog*)

Personally, this information was of more than just academic interest. I had come so far with experiment and direct experience, through trusting the wisdom of ancient traditions and healers to guide me. I knew what a difference a change in my feelings made to the world about me. Yet the rational part of my mind was still stuck in what I was beginning to perceive was an old way of thinking, born of an education that needed to be renewed in a fast-changing world.

Fortunately the doors are all open. We live in an age of dramatically expanding knowledge that rapidly becomes available to non-specialists. I needed to learn from scientists to overturn the certainties that had defined me as having a brain tumour. I wanted to be healed. Surgery was undesirable at best, or impossible. So therefore I was stuck unless I could find a way to change what my doctors and everyone else, other than the healers around me, perceived as a physical reality.

Understanding that the most advanced scientists were working with matter as something essentially fluid was tremendously exciting, the more so because the world it described reminded me so strongly of the unexplained experiences I'd had when I trusted my intuition. When Chad Orzel talked of quantum physics as a 'world where distant objects are connected in strange ways', my mind echoed with thoughts of people who could apparently communicate with a long-dead herbalist. Virtual particles 'popping in and out of existence' corresponded in my mind with the way I had found that something intensely imagined could become a tangible reality that everyone could see.

Most exciting of all was the fact that this world of quantum physics corresponded with the language of ancient understanding about the nature of the universe. It described an 'inner reality' that lay behind the physical laws of matter just like the inner world revealed by the intuition of mystics and available to each one of us. Though the methods might be entirely different, I found it was no longer necessary to choose between the 'truth' of mysticism and the 'truth' of science. The two reinforced each other.

A Hindu Vedic text composed around 250 BC defines our existence this way:

> The ultimate or irreducible reality is 'Spirit' in the sense of Pure Consciousness from out of which, as and by its power, Mind and Matter proceed. There are no degrees of difference in Spirit. The spirit which is in man is the one Spirit which is in everything and which, as an object of worship, is the Lord or God. Spirit is infinite and formless. Mind and Matter are finite and with form. Spirit is unchanged and inactive. Its Power is active and changes in the form of Mind and Matter. (Arthur Avalon, tr., *The Serpent Power*)

If I substituted the word 'space' or 'invisible quantity' for 'spirit', I would have what science has observed as constituting 96 per cent of the universe: dark matter, or non-atomic structure. If I substituted the word 'thought' for Mind and 'tangible or measurable objects' for Matter, I would have in this description something that corresponded not only to the world of quantum physics but also to the various different levels of reality I had begun to experience.

According to this teaching, Mind is essentially unconscious but becomes conscious in man 'to enable man to have finite experience'. In other words, we invent the separation between ourselves and the outside world to enable us to cope with day-to-day existence. Nevertheless, this is not the essential nature of our minds, which can expand beyond the limitations we have set. The essential nature of our minds is as part of the infinite, formless, pure consciousness of Spirit which is in everything.

These are difficult ideas to get a hold of in any practical sense, but perhaps it is enough to know that when you are struggling with physical symptoms or difficult emotional circumstances, what you see as a fixed 'reality' can change in a physical and tangible sense when you perceive it from a different angle or with another mental approach. When I am thinking about this, I often hear the poetic genius of Shakespeare and those lines from *Hamlet* ringing in my head:

> *There's nothing either good or bad*
> *But thinking makes it so.*

As I was readjusting my ideas about the nature of matter and possibility, I joined one of Martin's four-day classes teaching his healing method. Martin devised this course after his own healing. He had come to believe that *anything can be healed and anyone can be a healer*. If someone somewhere in the world has healed the thing that you want to heal, then it is possible that it can be done. He also believes, as I do, that if he could heal the tumour that had paralysed him and cause it to disappear, then anyone – even, and perhaps especially, a child – can be a healer. All that is necessary is to have the intention to heal and to learn to understand and perceive energy.

Martin used his knowledge of computer programming to set about condensing and packaging the tools of healing so that it would be possible for someone with no experience of healing to arrive at his course on the first evening and leave, four days later, able to give people healing and make them feel better. He still teaches these courses around the world and it is hard to find a more powerful or better constructed experience crammed into four days. Martin's teaching turned out to be life changing for me.

The power this process has to change people's perspective on the condition of their bodies comes from non-verbal exercises, where even a beginner is forced to rely on intuition. People who may have spent decades discussing emotional problems give them up to the magic of an instantaneous perception. This is the power of *feeling* change, as opposed to talking about it, and this is the power of healing.

The more accustomed to healing you become, the more you get to navigate a non-verbal world of energy in which a human being has the ability to influence others. It is like an electromagnetic wave that we direct to others by our intention to see them healthy and happy. Who can say what this unmeasured quantity is?

It is true that we all recognize it when we feel it, much as we recognize love or comfort without needing to have it explained.

Martin has devised a technique of tracking energy by the ways in which it reflects colour back to the mind of the healer. A perfectly balanced body will reflect this energy with the unbroken colours of the rainbow: the vibrations of the separate colours of light when it is refracted through a prism. Where energy is absorbed, heat is created, and someone being healed will often feel intense heat coming from the healer.

When the healer seeks to focus on the energy that is proper to each different centre of activity in the body, then all the colours of his energy should be absorbed except for the one appropriate to that function. So a balanced root *chakra* will reflect only red, a healthy sacral *chakra* only orange and so on. Where there are other beliefs, feelings or memories that influence the perception of the healthy functioning of that *chakra*, then other frequencies of light or colour will be reflected.

So this method of healing allows both the healer and the 'healee' to translate the colours into language and so consider consciously what the energy of the body reflects back to them. Change comes from the power of feeling differently and thinking differently combined. When the person being healed recognizes the feelings the healer has detected, then both know that a valid perception has taken place. The healer performs the function of a mirror to the healee's consciousness. Hence the name Martin chose for his technique: Body Mirror Healing.

Once you are aware of tensions in your consciousness that you may have hidden even from yourself, you are in a position to change them. Often the awareness itself is enough to free you from the physical tension or symptom that accompanies it. The starting point of this system is that all physical tensions have their origin in a person's mind, embracing your conscious and unconscious awareness, consistent with the teachings of Buddhism and yoga. Changing your mind changes the condition.

My first experience of this teaching was astonishing. I could easily accept the truth that the physical form is energy and continuously changing. I could perceive this energy in myself and others and sense the effects when it was transmitted. I was fascinated by the logical relationship between well-known physical conditions and the emotions or experience they indicated. This was like the understudy (the body), who knows everyone's part, being brought on from the wings to become the star of the show.

Nonetheless, when I found myself working with a complete stranger, with the expectation that I would not only 'heal' him but also have to tell him openly what I could 'see' in his energy, I trembled at the thought.

'Just make up a story,' urged Martin. 'Say the first thing that comes into your mind. Children can do this!'

So I went through the process Martin had taught us, and then, feeling as shy as a five year old, I told this man what I had seen in his roots.

'I saw a concrete mixer and it looked like concrete underfoot to me,' I said. 'There was rubbish everywhere.

Your roots need to grow into the earth so that you feel secure and nourished. So I lifted a section and dug a hole directly into the earth. I planted you in there, so your roots could get down to the real earth. I don't know if that means anything to you?'

The man was an actor, dependent on freelance jobs. 'I'm in the middle of building a house,' he said. 'There's rubbish and concrete mixers everywhere. It's very difficult to have any kind of stability, and my work has dried up.'

The root *chakra*, we had learned, is to do with security: job, money, home, as well as your relationship with your mother. I made no attempt to hide my amazement. 'That's extraordinary, but that's what I saw. I trust you'll feel a change in your circumstances with more security soon.'

All the time I was also receiving healing from others and their power was palpable, even though many of them were beginners like me. By the time the weekend was over I was uplifted by the experience. I felt I had made a deep discovery and I would never again perceive the interchange between people in quite the same way as before.

My symptoms had diminished, and I believed that the tumour would disappear with them. I believed I was healing long before the evidence of the scan showed me that this was true. In fact, I just wondered why it took so long for the evidence to show up on the screen. But I accepted the disappointment of the early scans without changing my course. After all, I had no option. I knew by now I was lucky not to have any competing 'treatments' being offered to me any longer. If this tumour was to go, it would have to be my way or no way.

Four months after the healing course I was due for another scan. This time I was determined not to let the oppressive experience of lying in the scanner destroy my optimism. Instead of lying passively, I made up my mind to work hard. All through the process I visualized white light healing the tumour and countering the impulse of the vibrations from the scanner that were bearing though my skull. It was not that I thought the magnetic resonance from the scanner was actually doing me harm – it was just that these intense invasive noises somehow represented my submission to illness and dependence on the medical system.

The scan lasted for 40 minutes, so the experience became extremely intense. Every time the scanner banged and clattered I countered it with my defence. By the end it was a rhythmic exchange – a kind of dance. Without moving a muscle, I was echoing every beat, mentally chanting *I heal* to every clang of the scanner's action. I left the hospital feeling a triumph of sorts. It was the first time since my diagnosis I had been able to go through a scan without feeling overwhelmed by a bitter sense of despair.

Two weeks later my husband and I turned up at the hospital for the results. I had everything crossed that they would reflect the months of positive effort I had put into anticipating the best outcome. We were shown into my consultant's office, where all the scans were up and ready to view for almost the first time. He had one from 2003 beside the new one from 2005. The first thing he said was: 'It's much harder to see than in 2003.'

Looking at the radiographer's notes, he sounded a bit confused. 'The signs are contradictory. I'm not quite sure what that means. I mean, I know what it means but not what it signifies.'

It looked to me as though the tumour had diminished. It seemed to be caving in on one side. The consultant seemed relaxed. He said he didn't need to do another scan for a year. As we left, my husband said under his breath, 'That gives you another year to work on it.'

This wasn't the dramatic result I had wished for but it was the first time since my diagnosis I'd had any encouraging news. The consultant was uncertain. My husband was tacitly supporting the work I was doing. I was exhilarated, even though I knew I still had plenty of road to travel. At least now I had begun to enjoy the journey.

CHAPTER NINE

Believing Is Seeing

Thought is a physical process.

Henry Marsh, British neurosurgeon, St George's
Hospital, *Midweek,* BBC Radio 4, 26 March 2008

Little by little, by infinitesimal degrees, my experiences in dealing with this tumour and its symptoms were leading me to overturn the old adage 'seeing is believing'. I was beginning to understand the opposite: 'believing is seeing'.

It was not that I had become so crack-brained that I was refusing to recognize the evidence before my eyes. Of course I wanted the reassurance of the image I saw on the screen and the relief of the consultant's unruffled reaction. It was just that I was not surprised, whereas the original diagnosis – that there was a serious problem with this body of mine that I had previously taken so much for granted – had astonished me, as well as scared me to my core.

In June 2006, just over a year later, I went back to the hospital to see the consultant for the results of another scan. I went alone this time. My family had accepted my confidence and believed also that the danger was past. Mr Powell brought up a computerized image for the first time; the MRI films on light-boxes were now a thing of the past. It took some time to get a directly comparable image side by side with the scan of the year before, but when my consultant pointed out where it was, I felt a rush of excitement. The tumour had visibly shrunk. It looked like the difference between a full sail, a spinnaker filled with wind and pressing forwards, and a flat sail that the wind has gone out of. This was enough for me. The threat was gone and I felt I was healed.

My relationship with my body had changed. We had made friends, so to speak, and I had learned to understand its language. I allowed myself to listen to it, to search my feelings for an echo of the messages it was giving me. Then I would allow my conscious mind to focus the full power of its logic on the problem that my body was drawing attention to.

Problems were not meant to be ignored, tolerated or swept under the carpet. They were meant to be solved. I was beginning to enjoy problems, instead of fearing them. I knew that I was healing. I had energy. I no longer felt dizzy and sick, and I no longer had crippling headaches. I had no symptoms other than a crossed right eye, and although I was prepared to live with that, I was able to have surgery, as the hospital considered the tumour 'stable' now, to tighten up the soggy eye muscle so that my eyes realigned. I felt that I was healthy and, now that I had the evidence of the scan that showed me the tumour was receding, I considered that I had crossed a dangerous ocean that I would never return to.

I understood that what I was doing on a daily basis was having an effect on my physical state but I still didn't understand why.

I was in love with the process of healing and the scope of the human mind. It was a vast landscape that had opened up right under my feet, ready to be explored. I laughed at the memory of my three-year-old self, leaving my brothers playing cricket on the lawn of my grandparents' home, and running as fast as my legs would carry me across the pasture next door. As I scampered away from the adults, leaping over tufts of grass, I made a decision which still rang as clearly in my mind today as it had nearly 50 years before: 'I'm going to be an explorer when I grow up.'

As soon as I left school, I began to travel around the globe. I had travelled to Mexico, Belize, India and all over Europe. I had lived in Beijing, New York and Paris – enough countries to realize that I was an Anglo-Saxon abroad, and to want to put down roots in England. I had done so, and I loved my roots: my family, my children, my home, but my three-year-old self was sometimes restless. I had thrown my explorer's temperament into information, books and discovering people's lives that were different from mine. But now, here was an unknown continent right inside my head, a territory with secrets that would change the way people felt about their lives, and transform the use they could make of them. Here was something I needed to explore. It was as though my three-year-old self was retaking the helm and steering my life on some course that she had known all along. I was happy to go along with it.

I had begun to take on people as clients, offering massage and healing to resolve physical and emotional problems. In this way I was learning more and more about the extraordinary subtlety of the human body's language. I had discovered the Hawaiian tradition of healing touch that allowed me to develop a powerful massage technique and communicate with my client's nervous system. Rhythmic repetitive strokes revealed the fascinating links between extreme points in a living body and the way the body's inner engineering inter-connects with zones that contain feelings, memories and beliefs. My hands were able to feel the connection, like a palpable electric charge, between the tips of the fingers and hips, or the ends of the toes and the shoulders or the palms of the hands and the neck. These relationships are not the same for every individual. They only show if there is related tension there, so each pocket of energy tells a story. Massage is a silent conversation with a physical body. When I reflected back to my client what their body was telling me, we would both feel the body let go of the symptom it had used to try to bring the situation to its owner's attention.

When you come to understand the body's language, it's possible to read the owner's emotional story like a book. Unveiling that story to the person who has brought their problem to heal is often enough to clear it straight away. It can take as little as ten minutes. A woman came to me for half an hour, saying she couldn't afford a longer treatment. She complained that her right foot had been so painful for a year that she was unable to walk. Her doctor diagnosed *plantar fasciitis*, but the treatment had made no difference to the pain. When I held her foot I suggested the problem stemmed from a feeling of anxiety about her ability to support herself and maintain her home. In an instant her suspicion dissolved as she told me tearfully that she missed her husband. She had nursed him for three years before he died, so no one suspected that she found it hard to cope without him, but in her heart she felt abandoned and frightened. The problem with her foot had emerged three months after his death. Ten minutes later, she got off the massage table. The pain was gone and did not return.

Touch is a powerful healing tool, but a healer can go further and deeper by exploring the energetic body you carry with you. The route by which you arrive at a point of pain or disease is unique to your way of seeing the world. I had come to see that pain starts in the mind, and only later shows itself in your physical body. It was by giving healing, using only my imagination and my intention to heal, that I was able to see the extraordinary subtlety and complexity of the roots of tension in our bodies. I was able to go deeply into my client's picture of the past, and explore the vision through which they had created their present situation. It was like flying into their world, a world without limits of time or geography or logic. It felt to me like travelling with them into the land of their dreams, bringing with me the power of clarifying energy, sweeping away shadows, dissolving blockages and putting everything back in its right place.

I found the poetic language of each person's energy profoundly moving. A man who came to me having difficulty establishing himself in his chosen profession seemed, when I began to heal him, as though he was standing on a stingray, floating above the surface of the sea bed but not connected to it. I interpreted this as his sense of disconnection from the earth, as though he had felt that things that related to security – initially mother, but later, job, home or money – were not really anything to do with him. When I relayed this to him after the healing, he explained that he had been adopted, and this image reflected his feelings about his adoptive mother. He could see how that emotion had transferred itself to his approach to aspects of his security in later life: his job and his home. Once he had seen this, he was able to let go of his resistance to making himself feel secure. I helped him to see how, as an adult, he could forge his own direct relationship with the earth, bypassing the shortcomings of his adoptive parent, and develop a sense of entitlement, as a human being, to enjoy the good things that the earth delivers him. Shortly after this, he was able to settle in a new place where he has felt happy and fulfilled.

A woman came to me with a frozen shoulder that had resisted months of osteopathy and massage. The symptom pointed to tension over something that she wanted for her happiness. The healing revealed that this somehow related to her experience in the zone of her sexuality. When I pointed this out to her and referred her back to the time the symptom had begun, she understood that the pain had started after her decision, following a miscarriage, that she would no longer try to have a child. This decision made her sad, but, consciously, she felt it was the right one for her. When she understood, she was able to release the emotional pain and her shoulder quickly became fully mobile again.

Another woman suffered from type 1 diabetes, for which she took insulin. She came to me more in hope that I could help her resolve some digestive problems she was having rather than the diabetes, because she expected that this condition would be with her for life. The healing revealed tension at home because she had been having problems with her husband over money. It became clear that she had grown up acutely aware of her mother's sense that there was never enough money, and the need for money had split the family from her father. She remembered feeling guilty, as a small child, about needing or wanting things that cost money. She had developed a habit of rejecting her own needs and desires for what she perceived as her family's benefit. Looking at her body from the point of view of what I call her 'energetic intelligence', the unconscious intelligence within every physical body, this mental habit showed itself in time as a physical rejection of sweetness. Her body failed to generate enough insulin to move sugar into her cells, the condition known as diabetes.

I didn't see or hear of this client for a couple of years after the healing, but when I did hear again she was clear of diabetes, had moved into a larger home with her husband and was happy. The 'treatment' she declared, had been 'brilliant'. Of course, I am glad to hear that, but it is only holding up a mirror to the relationship between a client's physical body and their emotional history, rearranging the balance and praying it will stay that way. Whether it does or not depends on what they do next.

Healing doesn't always happen fast. There can be many layers to be unravelled and resolved before it can occur. I considered the problem of my own body's 'slow response' to my continued expectation that it was healing, and came to the conclusion that it was like a battleship. It was built to defend me. Like my best friend, it had protected me from outside stresses and strains for many years without any change in its functioning. I was grateful for that. However, this resistance to change meant that it was slow to manoeuvre when I needed to make an alteration in its course. I had needed to keep my focus on the new course and remain patient.

Your body is your history. Your earliest perceptions, even those a baby is aware of in the womb, begin to affect your idea of safety or security. Each person's reaction to the events they experience is unique. Sometimes your reaction to your history can be so dramatic, or the consequences so severe, that it is harder for healing to happen. A Japanese woman in her seventies came to me hoping the healing would make it easier for her to keep food down and digest it. It turned out that she had no stomach left. She had survived three recurrences of stomach cancer, but in removing the cancer the surgeons had removed all of her stomach, her spleen and bile duct, half of her pancreas and they had used most of the duodenum to fashion a kind of substitute stomach for her.

When I came to do healing on this woman, I perceived a great disturbance in her root *chakra*, under her feet, where her energetic roots connected to the earth. The picture was like a house of cards collapsing into bonfires and the place of safety was constantly retreating and being swept away from her. It turned out that she had been born in North Korea, during World War II, which was then occupied by Imperial Japan. Her father was away in China, fighting with the Japanese army. When she was three, Japan was defeated and driven out of Korea by the Russians. She and her mother and little brother were forced to flee from the advancing Russian soldiers with a group of Japanese refugees. When I described the picture at her roots, she remembered that terrible flight to Japan. Villages were in flames as bombs exploded all around them. Children and babies were a danger to the refugees. If they cried with hunger there was a chance everyone would be discovered by the Russians, so crying babies were shot. She remembered how especially hard this had been for her and her mother, because she had a rebellious ebullient spirit. If she was told not to cry, she cried more loudly. But it seems as though her brain got the message. The hunger signals from her gut were a potential danger, not just to herself, but to her family as well, so the needs of her body should be overridden and suppressed.

Until this woman came to see me she had never considered the connection between her earliest feelings about the danger of meeting her physical needs and her subsequent experience of stomach cancer. The experience of healers is that cancer cells can develop when a feeling is held in and not expressed.

I had seen enough to become convinced of the power that thoughts and feelings could have over a physical body, but I didn't understand why. I wanted to know more so I could explain the route I had taken and understand the connection between dispassionate rational science and the emotional discovery I had made. I wanted, also, to bridge the gap that had sprung up between me and my family and oldest friends, if I could. They were happy that I seemed to be well, but I became used to the guarded look of tolerance mixed with disbelief that would steal across their eyes whenever my conversation touched on the reasons *why* I was better. It was clear to me that they felt I had drifted into some mystic bywater where they could not follow. On the one hand there was what we understand to be the rational thought that underpins our culture; on the other hand there was the murky world of 'belief' where I now seemed to have strayed.

The more I read, the more I discovered that medical researchers have made discoveries in the last 20 years that harmonize to an astonishing degree with the intuitive wisdom of healing. Tools like the magnetic resonance imager and the scanning tunnelling microscope have allowed researchers to observe processes as they occur in the body and the picture presented of the body in action on a microscopic scale is far more subtle and ingenious than conventional anatomy.

There is a tension, almost a contradiction, between the way the body works on a larger, physical scale, which we are all familiar with, and the way it works on a hidden, microscopic scale. This contradiction is similar to the one that exists between the laws that govern matter on a large scale, like physical mass, friction and gravity, and the behaviour of, for example, electrons on a sub-atomic scale. At this level, the solid is fluid, subject to the influence of intangible forces. Contradiction is a part of the structure of existence and the physics of our bodies expresses this perfectly.

We are accustomed to a clear distinction between living and dying, but in fact the process of creation and death is going on inside us all our lives. The programmed death of our body's cells is a key element of our health. The medical term for it is *apoptosis*, a beautiful Greek word that describes leaves falling from a tree or petals dropping from a flower. To create, enjoy and let go is the process of living, even on a microscopic scale of biology. You can liken the way this system functions in your body to a process of forgiveness, where we let go of the abuses or injuries of the past, allowing new growth to create life afresh.

When you are seeking to change or heal a part of your body, it's thrilling to learn that you are in a constant state of growth and renewal. Old abuses *can* be forgiven and forgotten. The cells that die most rapidly are the ones exposed to the harshest conditions. So the single layer of cells that lines your digestive tract, responsible for absorbing nutrients from your food, lasts only a few days. Your skin and hair cells are exposed to ultraviolet light and so they only last about a fortnight. And your blood, which is pumped around your body at high speed and squeezed into narrow capillaries dies and is replaced at the rate of about one hundred billion cells per day.

Paradoxically, it is this process of programmed cell death that allows us to develop a healthy body. It kills off the tissue between fingers and toes during the development of the foetus, for example, and eliminates viruses and defective cells. Researchers believe that many diseases arise when something goes wrong with this programmed cell death. Autoimmune diseases and degenerative diseases of the nervous system, such as Parkinson's and Alzheimer's, have been linked to faults in this system and cancer cells seem to resist the process of death and disposal, resulting in the growth of tumours. Your body is designed to allow the continuous cycle of birth and death to flow within you.

The death of your body's cells is balanced by specialized creative stem cells that are capable of making the appropriate one of about two hundred types of body tissue. These regenerations are happening continuously in every healthy living body, regardless of age, so you can see your body as constantly growing and changing. You may reasonably ask why, if your body in its natural state is such a wondrous fountain of renewal, anybody ever grows old and dies. The answer, of course, is that I don't know, but the latest research indicates that there are some parts of your body that are as old as you are: the muscles of your heart, the cerebral cortex of your brain and the inner lens of your eyes. The same research team *speculates* that stem cells, which are already rarer in adult tissue than in the young, also age as we do and become less capable of renewal.

Even so, the limitations of age are heavily influenced by our expectations. In the summer of 2012, Londoners and television viewers around the world were treated to the sight of a Sikh man from south London running with the Olympic torch. What is exceptional about Fauja Singh is that he was 101 years old. He had retired from running marathons the year before, a <u>hobby</u> that he decided to take up <u>at the age of 92</u>. His example means, I think, that we can expect to see more nonagenarian runners around the world from now on.

Exactly how stem cells operate has been the subject of a tidal wave of medical research in the last decade. Doctors are beginning to use stem cells' regenerative ability in some remarkable experimental operations. In the year that I have written this book, stem cells from one person's body have been used to regenerate sight in another whose eye was damaged by an acid attack. Katie Piper has been able to use her damaged eye to perceive shapes and depth of field since she had a membrane from a donor's cornea stitched across the front of her eye. The growth of these cells in her own body was stimulated by another membrane taken from the lining of a donor's womb and a course of drugs to prevent her body from rejecting the donated stem cells. In another radical medical experiment, doctors from Cambridge and the British Medical Research Council have shown how animals can use their own stem cells to repair damaged parts of their body. They extracted cells from the nose lining of paralysed dogs and, after cultivating them outside the body, re-injected them into the dogs at the site of the spinal nerve damage. Many of the dogs were able to walk again, with support, after the operation.

Stem cells from the lining at the back of the nose, called 'olfactory ensheathing cells', were shown in the early 1990s to have remarkable power. They were identified as stem cells that could not only regenerate tissue but actually reactivate damaged nerve contacts in the body's central nervous system, where all the automatic or autonomic functions of the body are taken care of.

It is interesting that these cells are the ones that have been shown to be so powerful, because the researchers have used them in a way that matches the 'energy map' of the body exactly. The intuitive *chakra* map, which sees the body as communicating layers of energy, puts the nose in the zone of the root *chakra*, which governs survival and security on the psychological level and bones and the skeleton on the physical level, with particular reference to the legs. The first and last breath of life enter the body through this zone. Science is now illuminating the miraculous organization of the body that conventional biology has underestimated for so long.

No surgery, however sophisticated, can match the subtlety and ingenuity that already exists in the unconscious mechanism of our bodies. Your body uses about 300 of your muscles simply to stand upright. The mind-boggling feat that co-ordinates brain, nerves and cells with the exact precision required to take you up stairs is fortunately taken care of by your unconscious mind, the autonomic nervous system. This system is responsible for 95 per cent of the way you function. So long as it is healthy, you never need to think about it. But when something goes wrong, this is the place to look for answers. The questions that are key to everyone interested in healing are these: Can your conscious mind influence your body's autonomic functions? How is that done?

All the experiences that you have read about so far in this book show you the answers I found to these questions: your body expresses your mind, which includes your conscious thoughts but also your unconscious feelings. When you look for healing, you need to use your mind to help your body, and your body can also help you know your mind.

Many doctors, schooled in Western medicine, which has considered the mind and body separate, have nevertheless found that their clinical experience confirms this point of view. Deepak Chopra, working as an endocrinologist in a New England hospital, witnessed the success of the same treatment in some patients and its failure in others. It was this experience that led him to re-examine his knowledge, and ultimately to revisit the Ayurvedic and spiritual traditions of his native India, which regard the human body as part of an integrated energetic whole. He tells this story in his book, *Quantum Healing*.

Since that book was published, just over 20 years ago, scientific researchers have used radioactive imaging to observe the way the body's cells communicate with each other, and they are reaching the same conclusion. American neuroscientist Dr Candace Pert mapped the interchange between messenger chemicals in the body and the brain and ultimately concluded: 'My research has shown me that the body can and must be healed through the mind, and the mind can and must be healed through the body.'

Your cells perform the intricate tasks we expect of them by communicating with one another through chemical and electrical signals. The immune system's forager cells recognize which cells are ready for death and disposal, for example, when the chemical that is normally inside the cell wall, *phosphatidylserine*, appears on the outer side of the cell.

What researchers have uncovered is the exact mechanism by which thought or feeling affect your physical body as much as the chemicals we absorb from food and medicine. The way in which your cells respond to chemicals they encounter is controlled by a gate in the cell wall called a receptor. Cell biologist Bruce Lipton found that cells can *change their function* when their chemical environment changes. He studied cells that line blood vessels and showed that when he added an inflammatory chemical, these cells converted to scavenger cells, or macrophages, designed to rid the body of toxins. They would then bind to the molecules of the invading chemical that was causing inflammation and direct them to the body's waste system, dying along with their prey. They did this even though he had removed their nuclei containing their DNA, suggesting to him that it is the gateway, the receptor, that determines whether or not the cell is under attack and how to respond.

The cell gateways are activated by the right 'key', poetically enough. The keys are the chemicals, known as ligands, which travel through your body looking for a gateway which they can unlock. When they find the right one, they bind to it and catalyse a reaction in the cell, changing its shape or function, automatically preventing any other key from getting in there. Some receptor cells respond to energy rather than physical chemicals. When they detect sounds, light or any other electromagnetic frequency that fits, they vibrate and change shape.

These chemicals that create events in your body can be generated by the organs themselves or by thoughts and feelings. Medicine, as we know it, continues to make a distinction between practical and emotional information, but our bodies are too subtle to make such a distinction. Hormones are key players in our chemical messenger system and one of them, *oxytocin*, which promotes contraction in the womb after labour, has been studied more extensively than others because it was the first to be synthesized outside the body. It turns out that this hormone, now found to be just as concentrated in the heart as in the brain, takes care of the emotional aspects of birth as well as the practical details. It's known to speed up labour and stimulate milk production, but it also promotes maternal 'bonding', including learning and tolerance, and, to underscore its key role in regenerating the species, it enhances a woman's experience of orgasm!

Our hearts have their own intrinsic nervous system. The heart operates in parallel and in constant communication with the brain, but it can function independently. This is what allows a heart transplant to work. When the nerve fibres to the brain are cut, as they must be during a transplant, the heart can function in its new host by means of its own nervous system. All the heart hormones affect the part of the brain concerned with learning and memory, the hippocampus, so that the more they're produced, the better we learn. This lends a new meaning to the notion of learning something 'by heart'. Our language seems to understand the way our bodies work better than our science has. Experiences that our language and instinct know will 'gladden our hearts' stimulate the production of chemical messengers, *dopamine* and *norepinephrine*, that have been shown to make us more sensitive and responsive, better at learning and retaining information and more interested in sex. Low levels of these chemicals have been associated with diseases that affect the nervous system, like attention deficit disorder or motor neurone disease. Our body's chemicals are designed to make us clever, communicative and creative when we are in love.

I reflected on the time when I had been embarrassed by the word 'love'. I have been lucky enough to experience it in many forms through my life, but even as I began to explore the psychology and mechanics behind my illness, to hear the word 'love' used (as I thought) indiscriminately made me uncomfortable. It conjured a power which my intellect could not fathom, and I was suspicious of it. I realized that, for most of my life, I had understood the profound heart at the core of my being in only a very limited sense. I had never imagined that a happy heart could have an overwhelming, detectible effect on my whole organism.

Your gut also has its own intelligence. Digestion is taken care of by a self-contained engine room that serves the whole body. Your bowel contains a hundred million messenger nerve cells which connect directly to the emotional and memory centre of the brain. Your gut generates seven hormones aimed at balancing your intake and storage of energy and communicates with all the major organs of your body. When it detects there is enough food present to process, it sends a message to your brain that you are full. When the insulin level in your body drops, it can send a physical and mental message to your brain denoting hunger. However, your brain can override the gut's self-contained system, and frequently does.

When you are frightened, your brain sends a chemical to your adrenal glands to prepare your body for fight or flight. The adrenals release the chemical messenger cortisol in preparation for anticipated damage to your body. Cortisol helps heal damaged tissue and stimulates your immune system, but it also raises your stress levels. This raised stress level sends a message to the brain to release more of the chemical that stimulates the adrenal gland. If your perception of danger does not pass, because you habitually fear one event after another, you can find yourself in a vicious circle. These chemicals, designed to protect you from attack, are in overdrive and create acidic conditions in your bloodstream which actually *suppress* your immune system and make you more vulnerable.

This is just one instance of how an unconscious but habitual emotional reaction, *a state of mind*, can interfere with the natural inclination of your body to keep you healthy. Our emotions, past and present, have a strong impact on how efficiently these powerful hormones are produced. These thoughts do not have to be conscious. The organs and the muscles, as well as the brain, have a physical memory of your previous experience. It is as though the emotional reactions of your past have imprinted a chemical pattern on your body's cells, and you need to revisit these emotions consciously to change the pattern.

Anger, which may become as habitual a reaction as fear, speeds up your heartbeat, secretes adrenalin and depresses the function of your entire digestive system. On the other hand, breathing, deliberately and consciously, slows your heartbeat and stimulates the nerves in your brain and your lower body, loosening movement in your intestines, and speeding the discharge of waste through your bowel and bladder.

No one has yet shown why some cells in the body defy the smooth operation of programmed cell death and regeneration and create tumours instead. However, Dr Pert and her husband Michael Ruff studied lung cancer cells and found them to have all the characteristics of macrophages, the scavenger cells generated in the bone marrow that work to destroy toxins. They found the cancer cells were, in fact, macrophages that had mutated. Instead of destroying the unhealthy cells, they were now splitting and developing, creating a tumour.

What if these macrophages are trying to do the job they are created for, rid your body of toxins, but when they get to the site of pain they find they are faced with something indestructible, something that renews itself as fast as the chemicals it creates are destroyed? Something, in fact, like a state of mind, like fear, despair or grief? If your macrophages are intent on doing the job they were designed to do, would they not send for reinforcements or find a way to split and grow in an attempt to drive out this intangible invader, like dedicated fighters pressing on with the job but overwhelmed by the general's poor strategy? If feelings have a tangible chemical consequence in your body, and we know that they do, wouldn't this be a reasonable way for a dedicated servant of your body like a macrophage to behave?

Of course this is only a theory that has crystallized for me since working as a healer and detecting the presence of feelings in various levels of the person I am working with. I can have a vibrational influence on changing the feelings I find there, but only the person I am healing can allow that change to happen and encourage a different state of mind in themselves. My experience is that when you detect the feeling you have been harbouring and release it, your physical symptoms are released also. Your body's mechanisms want to protect you at all costs. Your existence depends on the awe-inspiring co-operation of everything in your body doing the job it was designed for. Your feelings can upset the harmony of this system.

I believe that we all know this at some level of our being. It's just that our education has encouraged us to think otherwise. When I developed a daily habit of slowing down and distilling my concentration suffi-ciently, I could watch some of the processes happening in my body, like a supervisor on a factory floor. It was clear that there were so many complex operations going on in my unconscious that my conscious mind – the person I *thought* I was – was like the tip of an iceberg. The smooth operation of the whole organism depended on each side listening to the other, whereas until I became ill, my conscious mind tended to believe that it was all of me, and take my body's functions for granted.

People who have a daily habit of contemplation or meditation often understand that they can exploit their inner resources and decide to do so before turning to medical treatment. In the 1970s, when the detail about how intelligence circulates between brain and body was still undetected, a retired rear admiral from the British Royal Navy called Ernest Shattock found himself crippled with arthritis. His right hip had grown so painful he could not walk more than 100 yards. Faced with an operation to insert a metal hip joint, he decided to try self-treatment first. A programme of physical exercises that he'd done for about ten years had made no difference, but the admiral had also been meditating daily for over 20 years, having learned the habit as a young naval officer in Burma. He felt that he could use his mind to communicate with his body.

Once he'd decided to heal himself, he set about it with the efficiency you might expect from someone schooled in British naval discipline. He examined the x-rays of the deterioration in his hip joint in minute detail, so that he could decide exactly which of his body's cells were not functioning as they should. He spent about three months devising an alternative way of operating that would remove the arthritic damage, deciding he needed first to increase the blood supply to the hips, then to order the white blood cells to remove the calcified tissue from the area, and finally to remove the lesions on the joint itself. Once he had his programme, he spent 20 to 30 minutes each day at the same time closing his eyes, relaxing his body and steadying his breath while he sent out instructions to the relevant cells to do this job. He describes the process, with all the details of his progress and reversals, in his book, *Mind your Body*. For just over a year he continued to spend time every day consciously directing and visualizing his body's cells engaged in each of these activities as though they were ratings on one of his ships. Eighteen months later, at the age of 73, he had no pain and no arthritis.

CHAPTER TEN

Letting Go

. . . On a huge hill
Cragged and steep, truth stands, and he that will
Reach her, about must and about must go
And what the hill's suddenness resists, win so.

John Donne, 'Satire III'

Sometimes on the path to healing you reach what feels like an impasse. The hardest part of healing is letting go of control. It's a delicate balance. You know where you want to go. You want, more than anything, to be healed, to enjoy the life and the body you had before your illness. And yet before you can get there you have to accept, on a very deep level, that things are the way they are and that you have somehow created this situation.

You reach, almost simultaneously, a point of complete helplessness and a point of power. You accept that, unknowingly, you have reacted to situations in a way that has made you ill, but in that act of acceptance you gain the compassion for yourself that allows you to change direction and pursue your restored health. It is as though you can see the child in you, needing love and help, but you can see also the greater environment that the child inhabits. The meaning of the child's life, your life, is to pick a path through this great landscape and learn, by dealing with the obstacles you encounter, how to be happy.

Rational explanations helped me to feel in control of the mystical experience that healing had brought me into daily contact with. I enjoyed exploring the science. It boosted my confidence and helped to keep me fixed on the path I had embarked on. It helped me also to reach people who were resistant to knowledge that seemed irrational. Undoubtedly, I was making good progress, physically and emotionally. I felt I could float on any wave and emerge on the other side, unscathed, still floating. In fact, my emotional landscape had grown gentle. The waves and torrents of feeling from the past that had once engulfed me were history. I felt more robust, self-possessed, even sometimes bored, becalmed, waiting for the next adventure. There is truth in that old chestnut: 'Be careful what you wish for!' As soon as I felt I had assembled tools to deal with whatever life threw at me, I was pitched into a zone that was way beyond my power.

In 2006, just as I was convinced that the brain tumour was healing and would continue to get better, I began to go through what was probably the worst year of my life. First, my publisher decided not to go ahead with the book they had commissioned. I was humiliated. Crushed by the thought of all the work I had put into the book now being rejected without explanation. I felt I had let my family down and the news made me miserable.

It had always been important to me to do things well. Rejection had been a perennial fear. Now I was forced to look it full in the face again. I could hear the echo of other big rejections I had experienced in my life. I was familiar with the way each one seemed to rebound from the one before, as though they created one continuous theme. It didn't matter how far apart they were. Intervening happiness and success was drowned out by the deafening roar of not being good enough.

Each time I had felt like a victim. 'It's not fair!' or 'Why me?' would be screeching voices in my internal dialogue. This time proved to be different, though.

I had learned to see the world I experienced as a reflection of myself, and so to take some responsibility for anything that occurred. When something unpleasant confronted me, I knew how to search myself for a seed of what was happening. I had grown used to two traditional Hawaiian practices for resolving conflict and difficulty. There was the practice of forgiveness that I had used in clearing old wounds, cutting the energetic cords that kept me and other people in my life bound in conflict that had reached across the years. This simple practice, that the Hawaiians call *Ho'oponopono*, means 'the clearing', and I had experienced enough of its deceptive power with myself and others to be quick to put it in action when it was needed. This new situation called for some deeper introspection, however: another Hawaiian practice that, like much of their powerful teaching, masquerades as a deceptively simple phrase.

I focused on the painful rejection that confronted me and asked myself, 'What is it in me that has created this?'

Sometimes, when you ask yourself this question, about a person who has been angry with you or an accident you have had, the answer comes straight away. You can see how you have laid yourself open for bullying by not having confidence in yourself, or to an accident by not being fully aware of what you were doing. This time, I asked myself the question and couldn't find the answer. As far as I could see, I had worked hard to write a good story that needed to be told. Then, quite suddenly, the answer came bubbling out of me.

A friend had invited me to a colour therapy workshop that I looked upon as a pleasant day out. Somehow the conversation strayed to various problems the participants were having. The workshop leader turned to a woman and said, 'What does rejection mean to you?'

As soon as she said this I had a vivid flash of myself as a five-year-old child, curling miserably over the rail at the top of the stairs in our home. I could see tennis rackets and cricket bats spilling out of the brown wooden cupboard on the landing, from a door that refused to shut because the cupboard was so full of sporting equipment that had nothing to do with me. I could feel a great sob stuck in my chest like a lump that would break my heart, and I could hear my mother's footsteps creaking on the floor below. She had my full attention because she had just told me that the event I'd been so excitedly looking forward to was not going to happen. I'd heard a plan for 'the children' to go to Gibraltar to stay with my father in the summer, and I had assumed that it included me. My mother had just told me that it didn't. Only my brothers would be going as it would be too much to expect my father to look after a girl as well.

Half-immersed in this remembered scene, I was kind of surprised to hear myself exclaim, 'I know what rejection means to me!' and relay this memory to the workshop. I was even more surprised to find the lump in my heart come back and stick in my throat when I told the story, so that my voice broke and my eyes filled with tears. Everyone encouraged me then to release the feeling without shame, breathing deeply until I was sure I had cast it away on the tides.

Unexpectedly, I had reached near to the bottom of what rejection meant to me. Since I have, it has never meant the same again. I could see what it was in me that had created the new rejection I had experienced. I could see how I had carried my fear of rejection around with me, always ready for it to get between me and what I most wanted. For those were the situations in which it had always occurred, never coming between me and many good things in my life, but always haunting me just when I was on the verge of getting something that felt deeply important.

As far as my book was concerned I had another reaction to rejection that surprised me – I was angry. Some part of me knew that the editor's behaviour was nothing to do with my book. I was being made to pay the price for a managerial reorganization dressed up to look as if it was my fault, because that was the publisher's only way out of our contract. In the past, the pain of rejection would have been enough to make me slink away and hug my hurt in private. Now

I was sure enough of myself to be able to examine my case and successfully fight my corner. I brought up the evidence of my editor's previous enthusiastic responses to my manuscript. I managed to extract payment of my advance and then took the book to another publisher. It was published by Frances Lincoln just over a year later.

So was this the rejection to end all rejections for me? Seriously? No. But it taught me a powerful lesson. It was useless to expect everyone to love me. Some people would love what I had to say and others wouldn't. I would do and say what was important to *me*, and if some people responded and others didn't, then I could choose to go where people wanted to listen, or refine the message. This has been one of the most liberating discoveries of my life! Rejection is no longer a *fear* for me. It is just a piece of information.

Around this time I read something which neatly echoed this new approach. It was a story about an American manager who would routinely ask his sales team at the end of the day how often their sales pitch had been refused that day.

'How many times did ya get knocked back?'

If they answered 'None', then he would say: 'Well ya didn't try hard enough then.'

Rejection, I understood, is what anyone who has anything to offer can expect on a regular basis. It doesn't mean that what you are offering is bad. It just means that people haven't understood it yet. If you believe in what you are offering, then keep offering it, trying each time to make your message crystal clear.

However, there was a far harder lesson on the horizon, one that led me to discover my limits and the small power I have to prevent harm, even where I most desire to. This was the drama that overtook our eldest child, our beautiful daughter who was now just 16.

Our poor daughter, who had bravely followed all the details of my illness, and tried so hard to support me when I collapsed, had no need to be brave or adult any longer, now that I was out of danger. She was consumed with her own struggles for social acceptance and self-confidence, and gradually it became clear that she had found what she considered the perfect solution to these problems – she stopped eating.

Our little family was in turmoil again. Our child shrank physically and mentally behind a barrier that we didn't seem able to cross, while we each reacted to our pain with alternating fury and perplexity. Her father rebuked her, her younger sister yelled at her, and I begged her incessantly to eat.

'Your food is toxic!' she would scream, and yet it was food her body desperately needed.

Here was a dramatic demonstration of the power of the mind to overrule the body, but it was one that I would have given anything to have done without. When someone is starved, the impact on the physical body shows first. For two or three months, she was delighted by her solution to all the problems of adolescence. The beautiful curves of her body shrank and disappeared. She began to wear jackets and dresses made for an eight year old. She spent hours admiring her appearance. I could barely bring myself to look at her.

But when the body is starved, the mind grows dark, and she became trapped behind the barrier that she had created. Her face grew long and sombre, her eyes retreated and black depressions would burst from her like thunderclouds in our midst.

'I wish I was dead,' she would wail. 'Help me!'

For months I lay awake at night wondering how I could help her. She went to see counsellors, hypnotherapists, dieticians, but nothing could penetrate the barrier of control that she had put between herself and food. I spent hours trying to teach her meditation techniques to calm the terrible anxiety that now haunted her constantly. She would absorb them hungrily and then forget them the next day. I gave her healing, rebalancing the energy I could see inside her that was pushing her natural appetites away. I told her what I had seen and how it was changed.

'What have you done to me?' she screamed, and ran away to rebuild her defences.

I knew that she needed her defence against me, in part. After all, I was her mother, and I had always known that part of her growing up would be finding a way to rebel. I used to wonder, ironically, what rebellion she could find that I would not accept. We had been very close, and I couldn't imagine something that she would do that would be unacceptable to me if she wanted it. Now I was finding out. Acceptable rebellion did not include starving yourself to death.

I knew that she needed to get away from me but I also knew she needed help. I wanted to let her go and grow up in her own way but I could not do it yet. Her adolescent mind was simply not equipped to deal with the emotional and physical consequences of what she was doing. No matter where I looked for help, there seemed to be no one else around who could give it to her. She would not accept healing, from me or anyone else. Although she looked like a walking skeleton, she was on the upper limit of what the NHS considered a case for hospital treatment. Apparently she would have to get even sicker before they would consider admitting her. When she went to assessment meetings, she appeared calm and composed. She was still able to function at school, shutting herself up in the library for hours to avoid socializing in the canteen. But her periods had stopped. Her beautiful skin was now yellow. Her hair was falling out. And we all knew that her fear of food was slowly killing her.

She passed her seventeenth birthday, thinner than ever and with all the avenues of assistance exhausted. Desperate arguments and high tension now dominated our family life, all focused around the kitchen. She needed absolute control of every molecule of food, and she regarded everything I did with suspicion. She talked about eating, thought about eating constantly, even dreamed about eating, but she didn't actually eat more than a carrot or an egg a day.

I was exhausted too. This battle was harder than anything I had fought. When my own life was at stake, I was in charge. It was up to me to persist to the point of success. When people came to me and asked for healing, I was able to give them the help they asked for. But when someone I loved so much was in mortal danger, I could only give her as much help as she would accept. While she was paralysed by her fear of change, I was powerless. When she looked in the mirror, she didn't see the sick skeleton I saw. She saw someone who was liberated from the burden of flesh, childishly free of the bumps and lumps of adult womanhood. At times, when she wasn't in the grip of depression, she felt curiously ecstatic, as though she had achieved for herself what no ordinary person could.

I was in a place of despair, beyond thought. I took the dog for a walk and in the middle of an empty field, I howled out my desperation.

'God! Please, God!' I screamed at the clouds, 'Help me, please. Show me how I can help her!'

I had come to understand a great deal about a human being's ability to overcome physical limits with their mind. I had grown familiar with the power that one human being has to change physical energy in another human being. I had felt the mystery of the sense that my life was part of a greater whole. I had read about the divine and heard people talk about the divine, but I didn't really believe in God. I didn't have confidence that there was anything out there that would respond to my direct appeal. The voice that came out of me was from the childish depths of my soul, like laughter or a scream.

I calmed down, dried my tears and walked slowly back. On the way home I had an idea. Indoors, I put it to my daughter.

'If I were to cook you one of the dishes you used to eat as a child, and we weighed every single ingredient and calculated the calories exactly, so that you could be absolutely certain how many calories there were in what you were eating, would you eat it?'

To my astonishment, she simply answered, 'Yes.'

Later that day, I cooked a lasagne. She ate it. And the next day, she ate again. As the weeks and months went by she kept on eating. There were many problems for her to deal with as a consequence of her body's natural rhythms having been so disrupted, but now at least I knew she wasn't going to die.

So this is what they mean by prayer. I had no doubt that my 'idea' was a direct consequence of my passionate conversation with the clouds. It was a lesson for me that I knew was long overdue. In my stubborn discovery of my own strength, there was one thing I had overlooked. There is a power in this universe that is greater than all of us and yet it responds to the feeling in our hearts. I do not know what it is or pretend to understand it. But after this episode I began to use prayer in times of need, knowing that it would work. It has never failed me.

Every culture has a word for the power that is greater than mankind and yet interacts with a single man or woman. The Hindus call it *prana* and say that *prana* is on our side. *Prana* comes directly into us from the great amorphous creative space that is the essence of everything, because it is what animates our minds and bodies. Without it we would never have survived as a species. The Hawaiians put man's superconscious abilities at the crown of the head and rub herbs on a baby's skull to keep the fontanelle, the soft spot on the top, *open* for as long as possible. They say that the superconscious aspect of us can communicate with the Divine, but that we will never understand it. For a human to try to understand the Divine is, they say, like a dog trying to understand what it means to be human.

I looked to my dog and began to learn from him. He offered me devotion, and in return I would do anything in my power to keep him safe and happy. Devotion was an unfamiliar feeling for me, but it grew from a feeling of gratitude that, in some mysterious way, my natural environment, earth and sky, responded to my heartfelt desires. The more I was aware of the small space I occupied in the natural order, the more the natural order seemed to lend me its strength.

This 'acceptance', of my own limitations, of my tiny place in the greater scheme of things, of being a small echo of a greater sound that I needed to stay in harmony with, was for me the ultimate lesson. I understood that this was the key to prayer: letting go.

When my own emotions were entangled, all I could do was look for the part in me that echoed the distress I saw and release that. Again and again, I found that resolving the part that I played in events, however tiny, and offering this resolution up with hope but without expectation, had results beyond any I could have imagined. Again and again, my link with my daughter was showing me how this worked.

One night I woke suddenly with a clear head at 2.30am. It was a time of another family crisis. The day before, our daughter had telephoned our home in Kent from Thailand. Eighteen years old now, with no experience of travelling alone, she had just had all her money stolen and had also been turned out of the project in Pattaya where she had gone to volunteer. We had sent her some more money but beyond that we had no idea how to help or protect her. She was miserable, vulnerable and a very long way away. When I woke that night I knew instantly that I had to go and meditate.

I got up and went to the special corner I have for meditation. Our daughter's problems were at the forefront of my mind. In my meditation, I summoned the Buddhist image of Tara, the beautiful woman who embodies the essence and power of compassionate love. Once her image was clear in my mind, I asked her to take care of my daughter. In my mind I 'gave' her to Tara. I rolled my connection with my child out of the 'mother' in my root *chakra* and saw Tara accept this red ball of energy into herself. I understood that she would look after my child when I no longer could. The image was crystal clear and I finished the meditation and went back to bed and sleep.

The next day I spoke to our daughter on her mobile.

'Mum, you'll never guess what happened! I was on the bus to Bangkok this morning and I met this woman. Mum, she was so lovely! She was a Thai woman, about your age, but she was so kind to me. She started talking to me and, I couldn't help it, I cried on her shoulder and told her the whole story! She bought me a meal and lent me some money and then she told me to go to this monastery in Bangkok, and that's where I am now. They are going to let me stay here.'

'That's wonderful, darling. I'm so glad you're safe. When did you meet this woman?'

'On the bus from Pattaya to Bangkok. It left at 9.30 this morning.'

I felt a tingle along my spine like a breath. Thailand was exactly seven hours ahead of British time: 9.30am in Pattaya was 2.30am in England at that time of year. I told our daughter about my night time encounter with Tara.

She stayed in that monastery in Bangkok for five weeks and began to learn the power of accessing her inner strength in a way that I had never been able to teach her. I knew she was safe and cared for. The abbot of the monastery took special care of her and has referred to her ever since as 'my daughter'. I also knew it was no accident. My prayer had been answered at the very moment it was made.

My daughter's suffering taught me like no other person's could that the help I could offer as a healer was ultimately beyond my control. I remembered a scene from our past as though she had unconsciously been trying to teach me this lesson all her life. We were standing at the supermarket checkout. I was six months pregnant with our second daughter, packing the shopping away and trying to keep an eye meanwhile on this jiggling, jumping three year old who I had just picked up from school. She had been chattering away incessantly about the important events in her nursery class as we did the shopping. At the critical moment when I was paying the cashier, she asked, 'What is prayer, Mummy?'

The answer seemed blessedly simple at the time.

'It's talking to God,' I replied.

Outside the shop came the inevitable follow up.

'Who is God?'

I still didn't know, but now I had personal experience of an invisible force that responded to me when I asked it to. Many people sense this force but have different names for it. There are also many people who refuse to address this force, because they do not have a name for it. I know that because I was one of them. Even so, when I was in desperate straits, I found the instinct to pray was deeply embedded in me. Quite simply, I thank God for it.

CHAPTER ELEVEN

Speaking Your Body's Language

The world as we have created it is a process of our thinking. It cannot be changed without changing our thinking.

Albert Einstein

In March 2010 it was nearly four years since I had been to the hospital for a scan. I had seen the tumour recede and my symptoms disappear. Both I and the doctors were content with that. I was still in regular touch with Martin Brofman, having taken on organizing the UK residential healing courses he taught that had had such an impact on me.

One day he asked me, 'Why do you always say the tumour has receded, not disappeared?'

'Because that was the last image I saw on the scan, and I like to be truthful.'

'Of course, but isn't it time you went and had another scan?'

The prospect of revisiting the hospital filled me with dread. It had been the scene of so much misery and fear I was more than happy to turn my back on it forever. However, once the idea was planted in my mind I recognized that it had to be done. I hadn't been consciously working on the tumour for more than four years. I was happy with the life I was leading, and more and more convinced of the power of healing, but what if nothing had changed in the last four years? What, most horrible of all, if the tumour had grown? How could I reconcile that with my confident statements about healing?

I had learned to understand the language of people's bodies as though it was a spoken tongue. Usually the energy I put into their healing and this language, reflected back to them, was able to make a clear change in them. Some problems sorted themselves instantly, and others came clearly into focus to help them get on with resolving them. People were able to see the connection between their minds and their bodies, even if they didn't understand it. I was able to offer the tools I had used successfully to help them work steadily on persistent problems to the point of success, but I had also learned harsh lessons about my limits.

It was wonderful when healing was able to make a material difference to people's lives, but there was the deep disappointment of situations when the effects of the healing didn't last and the symptoms of disease continued to develop, in spite of it. Each disappointment was hard. However much I have learned from failure, I still love success!

Nevertheless, I recognize that the language I have learned doesn't work for everybody, and you cannot learn until the language you are hearing 'speaks' to you. That's why there are and will always be so many ways of communicating with the unformed energy that surrounds us and is within us. Multiple faiths have different images for the way the human brain can connect with this energy, and each one can be equally 'real' and effective.

I have explored many of these different schools, delighting in my new discovery of meaning in even the most familiar of them: the Bible I knew from my childhood. The Hawaiian word for the invisible energy that we are part of, which the yogis call *prana,* is *mana.* When I understood this and began to work with it, it gave me sudden understanding of the delicious and desirable 'food' I remembered from the Old Testament, described as 'manna from heaven'. The powerful images from the Bible, like the Tower of Babel where they speak so many languages that they cannot understand each other, express a truth about the world we have created. The tribes that we adopt for support, projecting an idea of ourselves that matches the collective we have chosen, blind us to a truth that we know in our hearts. We are the same as each other, and deep down we speak the same language. For me the essence of this language is in our bodies and the energy that circulates within them. The language of our bodies doesn't lie.

When you visit a healer or a doctor, it's like taking your car to the garage. Whatever happens, the car is yours and you are still the driver, but something has gone wrong and you need an expert's insight. A doctor will diagnose a mechanical problem. A healer is likely to diagnose an emotional cause leading to the mechanical problem. A doctor may propose a mechanical solution, which may correct the physical problem but have no effect on the energy behind it. It can be an excellent emergency treatment, although it may also cause reactions in your body because it is a foreign element. Medical treatments that are considered 'alternative' by Western medicine, like herbal or mineral medicines, also work on this mechanical level. However, if you accept that disease reflects your emotional state in a physical form, then of course you have still not dealt with the cause of your disease.

A healer will give you an energetic solution, so the effect is like having your battery charged. If there is a fault in the connections in the battery, or if it has been low for a long time, it will need recharging, until you are motoring confidently in your life, in which case you are recharging all the time, and you need a healer less and less (although it's always nice!).

There is a satisfying logic on the mechanical level of our bodies which is complete – except that it doesn't explain 'why'. A healer will look for the answer to that question which explains how the perfect balance of your life has come unstuck. For some people, healing may be an instantaneous moment of complete clarity and insight. For most people, healing your body from a chronic symptom takes determination and persistence. Changing your mind is the key to lasting healing, and you need to find the language that you understand that will make you do that.

Many people don't want change. They prefer to see their bodies as mechanical. They simply want to be relieved of the symptom and go back to the life they had before it arose, like I once had. Being restored to balance without pain, fear or alteration is what doctors seem to offer, and people would sometimes come to me only when their doctors had nothing more for them. Whatever their subconscious mental state happened to be, I could see it in the picture I perceived when I began healing.

Once, I gave a healing to someone who said she was open-minded about whether it could help or not. Even so, when I began the healing, trying to engage with the person inside felt like squeezing into a lift when the doors are shutting. Neither the healing nor anything I said to her afterwards convinced her that her feelings played any part in her illness. She didn't believe that *feelings* have any importance in the world as it is. It quickly became clear that the woman I was healing could not share my perspective on life but saw her illness as a random biological occurrence. We were both glad when the uncomfortable experience of being temporarily joined was over. I guess that she quickly shrugged off the experience, but sadly neither medical treatment nor healing could save her life in the end.

When I look at the world I see that everything created by human beings has its origin in our feelings. Love brings two people together to create new human beings. Passionate curiosity drives people against reason to put money and time into a building or a painting, into creating a combustion engine, for example, or trying to find a way to fly. Logic is a useful mental faculty that protects us. It stops us crossing a road when a car is passing. But it is not creative like love. Our feelings enable us not only to live as we do but to live at all!

Deep down, we *need* to be happy, but often we don't know any longer what makes us happy or believe we can have what it takes. Our sensitivity to our own happiness has been obscured by years of beliefs about duty, by shame or by guilt. It has been schooled out of us by families and society because happiness is essentially selfish. Even so, happiness is a form of selfishness that we need as individuals and that society needs us to have. Happiness makes us the most sociable and creative people we can be and so it is the goal of our existence. It is, as the character Elle says in the film *Legally Blonde*, what makes us good citizens: 'Endorphins make you happy. Happy people don't kill people.'

Deciding that you cannot have what makes you happy can result in the decision that life is not worth living. The result of that can be a fatal illness. It can be difficult for some people to get in touch with their deepest feelings. The process may take time for any of us. When we have constructed our lives around one way of seeing the world, it can be hard to accept that another way of living or thinking can be equally 'real'.

The discoveries of modern quantum physics suggest that our world is as fluid in nature as the ancient teachers said it was. What scientists still don't know is how the fluid movement within matter on the microscopic quantum scale crosses over to the very different physical laws that govern matter on a larger scale. It would take something really subtle, imperceptible in form, to connect both spheres. Something that even sensitive sub-atomic measuring devices have not been able to see – something, perhaps, as subtle as thought.

The yogis taught that matter is created from the unconscious 'mind' or spirit that embraces everything. The ancient Chinese said that matter exists in the ubiquitous invisible field of *chi* energy. These and many other civilizations have believed that it is 'consciousness' or 'thought' that creates division and form out of what is essentially one universal energy. Through a long process of contemplation and experiment I had come to understand that the first words of the Bible express this: 'In the beginning was the word.'

Human consciousness shapes the power that is the essence of our universe in the form of words. The words we use to talk to ourselves, the words we use to each other, the words we use to describe what we see and feel. Our thought becomes a force with a definable effect, like gravity or electricity. It can be used to counter those powers or work in combination with them, but unlike those powers, thought is a force that we, as living human beings, are masters of. It is the tool we use to create a reality that we can survive and thrive in. If we did not have this capacity, our planet would continue to evolve, with or without us, but thought is essential to human existence. By defining reality, our thinking turns existence into an experience that we can cope with, but it *also* creates the illusion of a definable reality 'out there' that we play no part in creating. In fact, reality is continuously created by our thought. The physicist

David Bohm described very well the confusion that the ability we have to define reality with our thinking creates in us:

> the general tacit assumption in thought is that it's just telling you the way things are and that it's not doing anything – that 'you' are inside there, deciding what to do with the information. But you don't decide what to do with the information. Thought runs you. Thought, however, gives false information that you are running it, that you are the one who controls thought. Whereas actually thought is the one which controls each one of us. Thought is creating divisions out of itself and then saying that they are there naturally.

In most situations, words are the tool that we use to turn the force of thought into an active reality.

The word creates time and space. Without it thought vanishes into the continuous round of energy in the universe. Words are thought made tangible.

One of the more beautiful experiments of recent years demonstrates the power that words have to shape thought and so change reality. In 1987 a 43-year-old Japanese businessman called Masuru Emoto was struck by the mysterious power of some 'special' water he had been given to heal a pain in his foot. A short time later he came across this question in a book about the mysteries of science: 'Are there any identical snow crystals?' His curiosity about this and the nature of the water that had healed him drove him to set up a practical experiment to see whether he could find two identical ice crystals.

Six months later he and his researcher were able to isolate individual water crystals enough to get a clear image of them, and the results astonished them.

They didn't find two identical ice crystals, but they did see something else. The frozen crystals either formed beautiful regular patterns, or they failed to show a pattern at all. The beautifully patterned crystals came from water taken from unpolluted natural sources; tap water and polluted water didn't form any crystals. What they then found was that dirty or polluted water could be transformed so that it would yield perfect symmetrically patterned crystals when people *spoke* to it kindly. They have repeated these experiments many times and in many languages since.

It isn't even necessary to make a sound to change the pattern of the water's crystals. When a jar is labelled with the words 'love and gratitude' facing inwards to the water it contains, the most beautiful crystals of all can be captured from its contents. The water is not reacting to the vibration of sound, but to the vibration of *thought and intention.*

To see how the power of our thinking works in ourselves we need to develop the habit of listening to ourselves, of watching to see how we talk to ourselves and how this is reflected in the world we experience. Most of our thoughts have their origin in feelings because that is where, as babies, we begin. This is what it means to 'know yourself'.

By going back to memories that had feelings attached to them, I had found I could see very clearly aspects of thinking that had become familiar bedfellows in my present life. Once seen, it was relatively simple to replace what had become just a habit of thought I had carried around since childhood. I could see that I was still making decisions with the wisdom of a child. What I had felt then was no longer important. Putting the expectation of what I wanted in place of what I perceived as 'reality' created a better experience for me.

A healer's insight into your condition may reflect back at you things that you already know you want at some level of your mind. This is something that is familiar on an emotional level that you may have decided was unobtainable or impossible for you. You may have believed that your point of view was a universal 'reality', rather than your personal version of it. The better you know yourself, however, the more you recognize that you create your own 'reality' and it is a flexible concept. You are open to your healer's insight giving you a new perspective on what is essential, and what is not, for you to live the life you want.

When this happens, as it began to with me when I met Martin Brofman, I would go so far as to say that you will be healed so long as you can keep your mind on this path. Nothing has more power for your life than your consciousness.

Once Martin had raised the possibility of returning to the hospital to check that my brain tumour had gone, I found, as so often happens, that circumstances were nudging me in that direction. A woman who I had not heard from for six years, since I had first attended one of Martin's healing classes, suddenly made contact. We had bonded over matching brain tumours, both of them affecting one eye on the emotional side of our body. Now I had an email from her saying that her tumour had grown so suddenly that she was being told she needed emergency surgery and the affected eye would have to be removed. Luckily I was able to point her to a different surgeon whose operation left her eye intact, but I recognized the message in this incident for me. It was all very well to be convinced of the power of healing, but objective assessment was necessary. After all, the remarkable revelations of magnetic resonance images were where this story had begun. That is where it should end also.

I contacted my consultant and asked for a follow-up MRI. He agreed and the appointment was set for December 2010. As I was anticipating this scan with some trepidation, I began to review the lessons this tumour had taught me. It was a paradox.

It had taught me both the limits of my world view and also the potential power of my world view. It had taught me my power as an individual, the power to make the choice I want, and also it had taught me to recognize how small that portion of power is. The way I saw reality was subjective, dependent upon my emotional expectations, and when I changed those expectations, reality changed. Each individual is the emperor of their internal universe and, while I may influence the choices they make, I have no power to override them. Yet, as an individual, I have the power of choice.

I cannot override evil or tragedy, but I can counter it with the power of expecting the best from the world and its inhabitants. That is my choice, my small contribution to the beauty I perceive in life around me. My illness had taught me how profoundly important it was to know who I was and why I had made the choices I did. Only then could I change them to something more desirable.

Nothing that happened to me was anyone else's 'fault'. The authority to make the decisions I did was always mine and remained mine. So the tumour had taught me to release blame and that the process of lifting it gradually ushered in understanding, compassion, gratitude and love. It came without effort, and its power continues to surprise me.

One morning, not long before the scan was due, I ran from the centre of Eastbourne, where our healing course was being held, to the top of Beachy Head, propelled by an inner fire of energy as wild as the wind in my hair. I was streaming tears as I ran, with the image of my father knocking around in my head. He had been dead for nearly 15 years and my tears had nothing to do with mourning for his loss. I had no idea where they came from, but something seemed to me intensely sad. The image in my head was not of my father as I knew him anyway. The person I felt inside my head was a young boy, a frightened teenage soldier who had had the power of life and death suddenly thrust upon him.

As I came to the top of the white cliff that towers above Eastbourne, I found the brick memorial where old soldiers gather every year to remember their friends who were killed in the war. I felt my father standing on my shoulders. The spirit of this young man who would one day become my father was clearly there. Here, palpably, was his deep love and loyalty for the men who had fought beside him and who had been his friends and companions during five long years of incarceration in German prisoner-of-war camps. I could feel how they idealized this very cliff on which I was standing, their image of the perfect home that they were giving their lives to defend. And now I knew where these tears were leading. More than anything, I felt the bitterness of their sense of betrayal when freedom could not match the perfect image they had forged, when, as the German defences crumbled and they could taste the freedom that would come with the end of the war, their column of marching prisoners of war was strafed by American friendly fire. Companions who had fought so hard to stay optimistic during the hard years of incarceration were killed by the very forces that were supposed to be liberating them. It seemed, to this young man who was my father, that you could trust very few people after that. You could only trust the ones you knew were just like you.

Trust was at home, symbolized by these white cliffs where I stood. But did the country live up to the promise it had held when he was a boy? Did its citizens even understand how much they had loved and given for it? Of course not. This is a new life and a new chapter now. My father's fear and bitterness caused him to resist the natural evolution of life, and I had somehow taken this personally. It was over now. I felt that I had glimpsed feelings that went way back before my birth. Empathy was understanding, and neither the tears nor the regret mattered any more. I thanked my father, or my mental image of my father, for this brief vision of a different emotional reality. Gratitude and compassion melted away grief.

At the very beginning of 2011 I met my consultant to see the results of the scan I'd had before Christmas. He apologized for being late, explaining that he'd had some complications from surgery he'd had recently. I wanted to offer him some healing, and I laughed at myself, but I kept my mouth shut. We sat down together to search the computer image of my head he had in front of him on the screen. He looked hard. He couldn't find a tumour. Eventually, he said happily, 'Oh yes. That's it. Let's see. Five milimetres across and thirteen milimetres long. There's no blood in it. Nothing there to worry about.'

I felt a triumphant thud in the pit of my stomach, like a pool ball hitting the net. This tiny thing, the size of the tip of my little fingernail, was no more than a piece of scar tissue. What did the consultant think of it? Would he declare that this was a miracle? Would he say that he couldn't understand how this had happened? Well, not exactly. This charming man, on the verge of retirement, and dealing with sickness himself, has other things on his mind.

'Well of course we don't have the earlier image on this computer, so I have nothing to compare it with. I think we never knew exactly what it was, did we? But it was obviously some sort of *meningioma*. Well, that's it. I don't think you need to come back for about seven years. I won't be here then. I'll have retired. It will be someone else. Take care!'

I could have kissed him!

What Can You Do for You?

The pages that follow are a summary of time-honoured practices that I encourage you to put to use in your own life for their power to transform your health and happiness. They are drawn from different cultures around the world but each one would be recognizable to another spiritual tradition, because they have one vital thing in common. These practices allow you to tap the power of the deepest parts of your psyche. You gain a perspective that allows you to see your emotional and physical make-up as an individual, and how that relates to your personal experience and your inherited experience. In so doing, you recognize your spiritual nature and enhance your physical and mental power. You are able to align yourself with the energy of your environment and discover the part you can play in it.

This is a big claim to make for such ordinary and everyday practices as you see here, but wisdom doesn't stem from technology. Technical innovations that have made our lives comfortable and entertaining have tended to have the opposite effect. They distract us from our own resources. When we dig deep into those resources we begin to recognize the extraordinary power we have at our disposal, if we choose to use it.

Each of these practices will focus your attention on the unique contribution that you bring to the world at this moment. They will allow you to enjoy your body, your mind, your feelings – just being who you are. If you do them daily, you will discover the way you shape your life and why. Gradually this point of view will show you what in your life you have power to change, and awaken your deep love for what you do not wish to change. You will free yourself to make the choices you want, so that you create the life that makes you happy, and healthy.

Breathe: Learn to Relax and Regulate your Breathing

Your breathing has the ability to take you beyond the limits of the boundary that you call yourself and to show you the depth and power that your body contains. There are physical reasons why it does this. The intake of oxygen alkalizes the blood, while, as we have already seen, stress acidifies the blood. So, straight away, you will begin to see some of the benefits that the alkaline environment you create inside, just by simple breathing, brings with it:

- greater calm, because you learn to trust your own rhythm and not lose yourself in fears
- more clarity and better memory, because your heart rhythm slows and its flow of hormones is not interrupted by tension, sending information directly into the hypothalamus, the part of your brain where your ability to be open to new information and to learn is sited
- greater happiness, because your heart will be generating dopamine, making you more alert to your surroundings, noticing things you haven't seen before
- more focus, because you will be teaching yourself to focus on just one very simple thing at a time
- relief from physical pain and muscular tension
- relief from emotional pain and tension.

To Relax: The Fried Egg

This exercise releases back, neck or shoulder pain, and relieves panic attacks, sleeplessness or stress. You need to do this on a hard surface for it to have its full softening effect on your muscles, so don't do it on a mattress, unless you can't avoid it. If you get cold, lay a woollen blanket on the floor and cover yourself with another. You can listen to music while you do this, but it is best to talk as little as possible, abstracting yourself from the daily round for 15 minutes to focus on your breathing.

- Lie on the floor with your knees up and your feet positioned comfortably on the floor shoulder width apart. Don't allow your knees to meet. Become aware of the way each foot rests on the floor like a tripod, at the ball of the foot under the big toe, the little toe and at the heel.
- Put a book under the back of your head, near the top so that you can feel the back of your neck floating above the floor. Allow the muscles on the back of your neck to fall into this space.
- Close your eyes and rest your hands gently on your abdomen.
- Let your breath out through your nose for as long as you can.
- As the breath turns to come in, feel your ribs gradually lift and expand sideways as the lungs fill up.
- When you can expand no more, allow the breath to escape gently through your nose again. Imagine

a wave coming onto a sandy beach and rolling up the beach until it sinks in and disappears. Your outward breath is like the wave sinking into the sand. Let your thoughts and your body dissolve as the wave vanishes.

- Watch the breath turn and fill your lungs again. You can imagine yourself being drawn back into a gentle sea with the power of your breath. Feel it push your diaphragm down, lifting and expanding your ribs as you float. Imagine yourself sparkling on the crest of the wave, reflecting the sun's light before the breath turns and you roll up the beach again. Don't strain. Just watch the breath release.

- Continue to do this until you become aware of subtle movements in the muscles along your spine. You will feel your shoulders spread out over the floor like eggs in a pan. You can listen to what's going on around you while you do this exercise but don't allow anything to distract you from the central fact of breathing.

- When you are finished, roll your knees together to one side and curl up before coming slowly up to standing from kneeling.

- Do this every day for 15 minutes or so, when you have finished work or when you are ready to go to bed. You will find that you look forward to the richness of your relaxation and appreciate the changes it makes in your body.

Two Yogic Breathing Exercises

Yogic breathing exercises, *pranayama*, are the art of getting the *prana*, the special quality of life or energy, to move in ways that create change in your body. In these exercises, unlike the Fried Egg above, you are interfering with the natural rhythm of your breath, so you should go gently. If you find yourself gasping for breath or getting dizzy, then change the rhythm you are using so as to make sure you don't strain. Then work gradually up to a longer rhythm when you are comfortable and begin to experience the benefits.

Your commitment to these exercises demands that you make a space in your life that is just for you, in which you can selfishly focus your attention on you. Without trying, you will become more aware of the emotional undercurrents that direct your life, as well as being able to glimpse the fundamental clarity and strength that you possess. These exercises are best done alone, in a space where you feel comfortable and can resist being disturbed, by the telephone or anything else, for anything from ten minutes to half an hour each day.

The end result of this commitment, paradoxically, is that you will be able to give more of yourself more happily to others when the need arises. The first step to your new strength, however, is to take time for yourself.

Daily regular practice is important. If you are rushed in the morning you can do ten minutes in the morning and ten minutes at night before you sleep. This has the advantage of promoting very sweet dreams!

Alternate Nostril Breathing: Freeing Yourself from Judgement

The yogis called this exercise, literally, 'homage to the life force': *pranavajapa pranayama*

Today it's generally known, less poetically in English, as 'alternate nostril breathing', but I think it helps to remember what it's for.

This exercise has been called 'tying up the mind with the cord of the breath'. It has the effect of making you feel calm and clear, activating and integrating the imaginative and the logical side of your brain. When you do this exercise, it is important not to allow yourself any self-criticism. Judgement is so habitual to us, and self-judgment so ingrained, that we need a holiday from it, to release the capacities we would have if we didn't judge them out of existence. This exercise will give you a judgement holiday.

You will breathe through alternate nostrils and hold your breath in-between in the rhythm of 1–4–2. So if you breathe in for 4 seconds, you will hold your breath for 16 seconds and breathe out for 8, and so on. You can increase the length of the breath if you feel comfortable with it but do not change it in the course of a sitting. Decide before you begin, how many counts of breath you will do on each side and stick to your decision confidently.

So, to begin . . .

- Sit in a comfortable upright position so that you can be relaxed and not have to think about your body. It's a good idea to sit on wool, silk or fur if you can, to insulate your body from the magnetism of the earth. It will also make the space that you create for yourself in your home feel more powerful.

- Lay your left hand on your left knee with the palm open, touching the forefinger and thumb together lightly. The forefinger symbolizes you as an individual and your thumb the universe that you are part of.
- Close your right nostril with your right thumb and exhale through your left nostril.
- Breathe in for four seconds through your left nostril and then close the nostril with the ring finger of your right hand, resting the middle two fingers on your forehead.
- Lower your chin so that you block the air escaping from your throat and hold your breath for 16 counts while you keep your fingers closed around your nose. (You can use your heartbeat as a time counter – this will give you a nice regular rhythm.) Keep your eyes closed but imagine yourself focusing on a point between your eyebrows.
- Release your thumb and breathe out through your right nostril steadily for eight counts.
- Breathe in for four counts through your right nostril.
- Close the right nostril with your thumb and hold the breath for 16 counts, as before.
- Release the breath through your left nostril for eight counts.

This completes one cycle of the homage to life force breath. Repeat it four times if your initial in-breath was for four counts, five times if the initial in-breath was five counts, and so on. Make all your actions smooth and unhurried. If you are straining to keep your breaths even, reduce the pattern to 3–12–6. If you find it easy to breathe 4–16–8, then increase it to 5–20–10 the next day. If you are confident that you are keeping the right rhythm or if you can count and think something else at the same time, then repeat the word 'Aum' soundlessly to yourself as you do it. This word means 'all there is' in Sanskrit and is pronounced 'aaaaummmm'. The vibrations generated by the sound made internally are credited with balancing the individual body and mind in a proper perception of your place in the immensity of creation.

The Cleansing Breath, or Bhastrika Pranayama

This exercise can follow on from the one before, or, if you are short of time, you can alternate the exercises on different days. Of course, the more you do, the quicker you will experience the benefits.

It's a powerful exercise for calming fear and anxieties. While doing it you can imagine viewing yourself as though from the outside. As you do so you can see clearly what you desire and allow yourself to imagine that desire has been achieved. You can look forward to the day ahead as though you were getting ready to play a part on a stage. Prepare yourself to play it with enthusiasm and skill, whatever your fears at the moment. You can anticipate the applause and approval you will receive for it.

When you hold your breath in this exercise you can imagine that you are filled with clear energy that is constantly refilling you like a magic glass bottle. By doing the exercise you are learning to manage the energy in your body. If you have been feeling tired or sluggish and need to boost your vitality, make the last breath before you hold it an in-breath. If you have been anxious or nervous, suffering panic attacks or depression, breathe out on the last breath and hold it there while you count. You will find it makes no difference to how long you can comfortably hold your breath for, but it does have a powerful effect on your body and mind.

This exercise takes about five minutes for the whole cycle. Read through it once before you begin.

- Start by sitting as before.
- Place your hands palm upwards on your knees with the thumb and forefinger lightly touching together.
- Take 11 deep rhythmic breaths, bending the body forward as you breathe out, straightening the spine upright as you breathe in. After 11 breaths, drop your chin and gently stop breathing. Imagine you are sending your breath down to the base of your body and gently tapping a stopper on it.
- Hold your breath calmly for as long as is comfortable. Don't strain. You will find that if you relax when you want to release your breath or take more in, then you can easily defer it for

another ten counts or so. You can hold the breath for 40 counts, 60 counts and gradually extend to 70 counts. The more you concentrate on the breath, the longer you will be able to hold it comfortably.

- As you become more accustomed to restraining your breath, allow yourself to think forward to the events of the day and the things you would like to achieve.
- When you are ready, gently begin to take another 11 breaths and repeat the cycle.
- Do three cycles of this breathing.

You can do the exercise with 21 preparatory breaths in each cycle instead of 11. You may find you can restrain your breath comfortably for longer if you prepare with 21 breaths.

Your Body as Energy: Understand the Correspondence Between Physical and Emotional Feeling

When the map of the *chakras* is laid alongside a modern medical map of the body's anatomy, there is a striking correspondence between the *chakras* and the clusters of nerve endings, or glial cells, that lie alongside the spine, as well as the endocrine system.

The *chakra* system is based on the Indian Vedic texts of 600 BC. Until the modern age, all medical practices took into account the patient's emotions as a cause of disease. Chinese medicine identified certain emotions with particular organs, such as the location of anger in the liver, while Ayurvedic and European herbalists sought to balance elemental 'humours', creating hot, cold or dry conditions in the body. Of all maps of the body's energy, I have found the *chakra* map makes the clearest links between the physical and emotional aspects of your self and puts this in the context of your spiritual being.

These are the broad characteristics of the *chakras* that I work with, based on what I have learned from different teachers and traditions as well as the functions of the nerves and glands in the zones they cover. Referring to this chart can help you to see the correspondence between physical problems and emotional issues in your life, and also what you would most like to resolve.

Chakra: Characteristics and Associations	Balanced State	Out of Balance
Root: base of the trunk, legs and feet Colour: red Vibration: middle C (Do) Sense: smell Connection to mother and by extension to the earth Element: earth Develops from conception to age 2/3	Trusting Energetic Joyful Secure Generous Practical Good digestion/ elimination	Fearful Restless Hesitating Problems with elimination, bones, legs or feet; sciatica Insecurity Feeling poor Nostalgia
Navel: lower trunk around sacrum Colour: orange Vibration: D (Re) Sense: taste Appetite for food and sex Centre of emotion and unconscious physical memories Hawaiian: the Child Element: water Develops from age 3 to 6	Sensual Emotional Balanced Understanding Sociable Enjoys laughter Contented Source of healing energy in some traditions	Problems with genitals, reproductive organs Over- or under-appetite for food, drink or sex Low satisfaction from food, drink or sex Lower back pain

Chakra: Characteristics and Associations	Balanced State	Out of Balance
Solar Plexus: Stomach region Colour: yellow Vibration: E (Mi) Sense: sight Associated with sense of self, ego, will, power and freedom, logic and the conscious mind Hawaiian: the Mother (of the self) Element: fire Develops from age 6 to 9	Confident Clear sighted Strong logic Purposeful	Anger Shyness/diffidence/timidity Problems with eyesight/eyes Low energy – adrenal exhaustion Muscle weakness Diabetes or other problems with digestive organs in this region: stomach, pancreas, gall bladder, kidneys (see also root *chakra*) Over-analytical/literal
Heart Colour: emerald green Vibration: F (Fa) Sense: touch Associated with loving, relationships, breath and heart Element: air Develops from age 9 to 12	Loving Tolerant Open Compassionate Tactile Calm Content	Asthma; lung congestion or other breathing problems Heart irregularities High or low blood pressure Poor immune system Blood disorders Poor learning and memory (see also crown *chakra*)

Chakra: Characteristics and Associations	Balanced State	Out of Balance
Throat: includes arms and hands Colour: sky blue Vibration: G (So) Sense: hearing Intuition, self-expression Element: ether Develops from age 12 to 15	Communicative Imaginative Intuitive Instinctive Good hearing Musicality	Secretive Indecisive Problems with hearing, ears Hyperthyroid or hypothyroid Problems with throat, neck, shoulders, arms and hands
Brow Colour: indigo Vibration: A (La) Sense: psychic perception Spiritual connection, sense of mission, purpose in life Develops from age 15 to 18	Self-possessed Motivated Wise	Poor balance Poor memory Pituitary gland problems Hormonal imbalances Self-critical (as also heart)
Crown Colour: violet Vibration: B (Ti) Sense: union with environment Connection with father and authority, and to the Divine Hawaiian: the Superconscious (the Father) Develops from age 18 to 21	Connected Guided Aware Peaceful	Isolation Arrogance Poor relationship with authority Nervous disorders: Alzheimer's, Parkinson's, meningitis Hair loss

Old Wounds Meditation: Learn How to Release your Feelings Without Harm

Buried feelings can be immensely destructive, shaping the way you behave and the way the world reacts to you. Most of the time you can be quite unaware of them, but occasionally they emerge from their hiding place and turn everything upside down. Even then you may not want to let them go. Our feelings can feel like ourselves. It often seems that if we let them go then we are reducing ourselves to nothing. Even so, once you try it, you will find that releasing your feelings brings you energy and creativity as well as freedom from pain. Old feelings are part of the baggage you will find it easier not to carry with you in your life. These simple methods have powerful potential to help you release what you don't want.

Self-Healing Meditation for Old Wounds

When you try to do something simple or peaceful, like breathing or meditation, and you find you cannot, it is almost certain to be because you have undercurrents of emotion playing on your mind. Those feelings are shaping your life daily. If you find you are in trouble, with either physical problems or a difficult mental state, then this is a great way to unravel what has gone wrong. The 'old wounds' meditation will allow you to look inside yourself and see clearly the decisions you have taken in the past. You can do this by yourself, or work with a healer or someone you trust to have your best interests at heart. You may be able to go deeper with someone else to support you.

For this healing you allow yourself to slip into a relaxed physical and mental state and trust your imagination. When your breathing is relaxed and slow, and you are not trying to think, your mind is working at its strongest rhythm, the alpha rhythm. You allow yourself to feel, rather than think, because you may have imposed restrictions on your feelings at the level of logic, and this exercise is designed to show you feelings you have kept hidden from yourself. As a result, it is faster and more effective than hours of talking about a problem can be.

Start by deciding to set aside a time in your day for you alone, half an hour each day when you sit quietly in a place where you feel safe and where you won't be disturbed. Have a glass of water near you and a notebook where you can scribble down thoughts that come up. The water will help you put a distance between yourself and the old feelings when you have completed the process, and the notebook will make sure you don't let your earliest impressions slip away.

Now you need to relax your body completely. As you grow accustomed to doing this every day, you will find you can reach this meditative state of relaxation very quickly. At first, relaxing into yourself may take ten minutes or so, or you may prefer to do it with a recorded relaxation guide.

- Make yourself comfortable, but not so comfortable that you fall asleep! Sit or lean upright as this helps to focus. Lay your hands palms upward on your knees.

- Close your eyes and take a deep breath, letting your diaphragm collapse as you let the breath go. Mentally tell yourself to relax.
- Take another deep breath and let it go, giving yourself the instruction 'Relax'. As you do so imagine a ball of white light sitting in the palm of each hand.
- Take another breath. Let it go. Imagine these balls of white light travelling up your arms, into your shoulders, throat and chest.
- Now send the ball of white light up into your head. See it relaxing each part of your scalp, forehead, eyebrows, nose and jaw as it touches them.
- Send the light down your body, telling your lungs, internal organs, legs, feet and toes to relax. Feel them doing so.
- Now imagine yourself in your favourite place, by the sea, in a garden, in a deep green wood or a tropical forest. Put yourself there and smell the air, hear the rustle of leaves, feel the wind on your face or the sun on your skin. Enjoy these sensations for a minute or so.
- Then, in your mind, count down: 3 . . . 2 . . . 1. When you reach 1 you will see the number like a door before you. Imagine walking towards this door and pushing it open.

On the other side of this door is your earliest memory.

If you can remember anything before the age of four, you are in the root *chakra*. The colour of the world around you is red.

Concentrate on this first memory and allow yourself to be the child at the centre of this drama. What is happening and what is it making you feel?

Who else is in the picture? Where is your mother? What is the relationship between you?

Allow yourself to express your feelings to your mother in your mind's eye, bringing her forward so that she can hear you speaking.

Now, listen to her response. Wait until you have a clear idea of what she is saying. Continue to express your feelings without restraint and listen to her response until you feel there is nothing left to be said.

When you are ready, let her go. Imagine that she has turned into a big red helium balloon and is rising above the horizon. As she drifts away from you, take a big pair of imaginary scissors and cut the string that binds her to you. See her float over the horizon and disappear.

Come back into the sense of your own body in the present. Become aware of how you are sitting, and of how the ground or the chair you are sitting on relates to the earth. See if you can feel the energy of the earth beneath you and around you, seeing yourself as part of the red vibration of its energy. Imagine roots coming from the base of your body going down deep into the earth, releasing emotional and physical waste on one side and bringing up new creative energy from the centre of the earth into your body on the other side.

Understand that the earth is always ready to absorb your weakness and continually renews your strength, because your strength is an expression of the earth's energy. Relish the feeling of safety that this gives you and express your gratitude to the natural order if you feel moved to do so.

Now gradually begin to move your fingers and toes and muscles, while allowing this feeling of safety to spread through your whole body. When you are ready, open your eyes, take a sip of water, and reflect on the experience. Note down any intense feelings that have arisen and allow yourself to reflect at leisure on the relationship of those feelings to your current life.

The root *chakra* mirrors your experience of being nurtured by your mother, both in the sense of the way she nurtured you and your individual reaction to that. As it is the most fundamental *chakra* of life, it embraces everything to do with security and survival. In your adult life, therefore, it relates to job, home and money. Trust, or the lack of it, fear, is also founded in the root *chakra*.

Was there conflict with your mother? Did you reject her care? Or did you have a good relationship with your mother but also adopt her fearful attitude to security? There is a myriad of possibilities contained in your mind's memories, and you will probably quickly see how they have shaped your life now.

Does your current experience of security, money or job reflect the emotional reaction you have just remembered? If you had to put your reaction into words, what would they be? Can you imagine different words that describe a situation you would like?

What if you cannot remember anything in your life before the age of four? Still go back to your earliest memory when you begin the old wounds healing. You will see from the guide in the chart which aspect of your life it relates to. Revisit the memory in exactly the way described above. The only difference will be in the colour of the environment you imagine, and the aspects of your life that have been affected.

Explore the memory in your meditation. Whatever your feelings, do not be afraid of them. Nothing that happened then can reach you now. You have survived all the hurts and accidents of your past. The person who hurt you was passing on their own pain. Say what you want to say to the other person or people involved. Explain how you felt. Scream or shout at them in a way you weren't able to at the time if you need to. Your emotion will do them no harm now, but it is something you need to release. Do not judge the feelings that you uncover. Just allow them to emerge and look at them as any adult might look compassionately on a child.

Remember always to wait and listen to the other person's response when you ask them why they did what they did to you, and continue until there is nothing left to be said on either side. You will understand why they treated you as they did. Their words and actions will no longer hurt you.

Accept that you have grown beyond the pain you felt then. You are healing yourself, and you can leave this pain behind.

Remember also to release the person from your memory when you have finished. See them ready to leave when all the hurt or anger is gone. When you are ready, take your imaginary pair of scissors and let them go – imagine them floating away over the horizon like a colourful helium balloon.

You can return to a *chakra* in meditation as many times as you like if you feel there is unfinished business. As you release old feelings that you have held in this part of your body you will feel a new sense of understanding and strength. As you deal with one memory after another, you will find that earlier memories emerge. Treat them in the same way until you have reviewed your attitudes to all the things that matter most in your life in this way.

If there is one *chakra* that is a blank, then you can use your imagination. You can put yourself in the position of a conscious spirit *imagining* the relationship between your mother and father at the time of conception, for example. What were the hopes and fears of each of them, and, assuming that you had a choice, why would you have chosen to be born into this relationship? What has their relationship taught you or given you?

Earth Healing

If you have delved into feelings that you have kept carefully stored away, you may have unleashed powerful passions. Intense memories bring feelings with them like waves. When you first uncover the memory, the emotion associated with it wells up inside as fresh as the day it occurred. Sometimes intense feelings come upon you without warning and apparently without reason. Or perhaps you just feel physical pain. In any case, you need a quick fix for overwhelming feelings and pain. This exercise enables you to release physical and emotional pain. You will come to see yourself as a cork, capable of floating indestructibly over great waves of feeling.

People often ask me, 'How do I stop this feeling?' It's as though feelings have some independent reality that has taken possession of us. But you have a creative mind that can overwhelm painful feelings and accessing it is easier than you think. I developed this five-minute fix to deal with emotional shocks that came up like tidal waves within me when I began my healing. When I was suddenly consumed by intense anger or fear, it would feel as though I was about to drown. This is what happens when you have a panic attack. If you cannot find the feeling and let it go, then the next fear you put in place is fear of the panic attack itself. We build up layers of fears so that the original cause is buried. Doing this exercise not only helps to release the layers one by one, but gets you through the storm of intense physical or emotional pain. You will find you release new energy and a fresh outlook, as well as an ability to deal differently with the people in the present who are still attached to pain from the past.

It is best to do this outside, where you can be out of sight and unselfconsciously free. You need to make your own private connection with the magnetic earth that you come from, and as you develop this personal communication with the earth as your 'mother', you will discover an immense, inexhaustible source of strength and support in your life.

It would help you to bear in mind that our parents give us life, but on a grander scale of things it is up to each individual to develop their own relationship with the universe during his or her lifetime. On this scale, the earth supplies all our needs as human beings. Everything that we have or use comes from the earth in the first place and goes back into the earth when we are finished. It is a continuous benevolent cycle in which we play our part by recognizing the bounty of the earth in the form of our lives, our food and our raw materials, while we use our creativity and ingenuity to transform these things. When we have finished we give the waste back to the earth again, where it is transformed once more into something usable. Everything we need depends on this benevolent cycle. When we are aware of how much it works in our favour, we strengthen our relationship with our home, our job and money as we develop a trusting relationship with the earth to supply our needs.

This process also works with our feelings. They come from our experiences, lodge in our bodies, effecting changes and mutations, but they can also be consciously identified and given back to the earth in the way described below. This is what it means to feel 'rooted'. It is not necessarily to stay in the same place, keep the same job or house, but to know that you can get benefit from the earth as a human being wherever you are. You receive nourishing energy from the earth and it is your privilege to give negative energy back, instead of carrying it around with you, as though the earth were your ideal mother. Letting go of your feelings makes you more receptive to earthly energy in your present space. You become aware of how you are part of the 'flow' of your environment.

So to begin . . .

- Stand, in shoes or bare feet, in the open if possible. Your feet are facing forward, shoulder width apart, your knees slightly bent and your arms relaxed by your sides. Close your eyes.
- Breathe out for as long as you can through your nose, and then fill your lungs, feeling the base of your ribs widen as the breath fills you. Watch the tide of breath turn smoothly, like a wave running up the beach and flowing back again. Do this three times.
- Feel the toes of your right foot (left foot if you are left-handed) sink into the earth's skin, the outer edge of the foot, then the ball of the foot, the heel of your foot, with the line between them which is the mirror image of your spine. Do the same with your other foot, so that you feel both feet are properly planted.
- Greet the earth under your feet. It's better if you speak aloud because the act of speaking engages your unconscious more fully and focuses your will. Say, for example:

    I greet you earth mother and I ask you to accept all the tension, pain and wasted energy in my body. I give you my fear, my impatience, my anger, my negative feelings, and I ask you to accept them into yourself. Thank you.

- Consider the feeling that you wish to be free of. There is little difference between physical and emotional pain, so this will work for either. As you think about your feeling, you will be able to locate the part, or parts, of the body where it is centred. Imagine that you are rolling up the pain like a bundle of waste paper until it is a concentrated ball that you can roll down your body.
- Imagine yourself rolling this bundle down your right leg (left leg if you are left-handed) and watch it in your mind as it travels through your foot into the earth's skin, through her rocky muscles, her dark caves and tunnels, her subterranean seas and into the fiery heart which is the energy at her core. Watch the earth's fire destroy all the waste you have entrusted to her. Focus completely on your right foot (left foot), allowing your weight to shift from your left (right) so that it feels 'empty'.
- Now return your balance to the centre. Imagine the white-hot energy from the earth's core running back up through the layers of lava and rock, soil and plants beneath you. Feel it come up through the sole of your other foot, through the bones and muscles of your calf, into your knee and thigh, until it reaches the point at the very base of your spine. See this bright ball of energy kindle at the base of your body into a red glow and allow it to rise up through your entire body.
- Breathe in slowly through your nose and gently let the breath go. Imagine yourself putting down

roots that run down your legs and deep into the earth.

• Check the original site of the pain you felt and see how it feels now. Note improvements and any feelings or memories that occur to you as you do this. Thank the earth for her care and protection.

Forgiveness

There are only two kinds of forgiveness . . . Now or Later.

Kumu Harry Uhane Jim

Some things that people have done seem 'unforgivable'. The sense of betrayed trust is so deep that we feel destroyed by it. It's hard for us to accept responsibility for anything that has been so wounding to experience. Our anger and hurt can emerge suddenly, as if out of nowhere, like a sudden storm that sweeps us away from our course, despite everything we have done to let it go. Then we need some extra help.

Why should you forgive? Quite simply, for selfish reasons: it liberates you and allows you to continue your creative journey through life.

When you forgive, the person or people you are forgiving cannot play the game of guilt, shame or pity that, by not forgiving, you have obliged yourself to participate in. It is as if your hurt has joined you to them in a game of tug-of-war. As soon as you drop your end of the rope, the game is over, and you are free to choose the game you play. You no longer have to respond to the one that was thrust upon you.

To forgive is to take power. Forgiveness is the power of yielding, the *yin* or negative energy, used to overwhelm the power of aggression. This is the power a *T'ai Chi* master uses to defeat his attacker. A master yields when he is attacked, carrying with him as he retreats the full force of his opponent's energy. When this energy reaches the end of its force, deflected without causing damage, it can be flicked aside. This receptive feminine energy also creates revolutions. It was the power that Mahatma Ghandi used against the might of the British Empire. It is the power that was used by Nelson Mandela to build the foundations of a new South Africa. It is a power that will bring you to the centre of your strength if you use it in your own life.

When you view your life from a spiritual perspective, one that takes in the circumstances of your birth, the nature and character of your parents and the incidents that you have experienced, you see that you have been learning from every circumstance. Sometimes you have learned things that make you happy, sometimes the opposite. But you cannot avoid the learning. Once you have learned the lesson, it is time to let go of the experience that taught it to you. You have no further use for it, and if the experience has been unpleasant you don't want it in your life. Forgiveness will do this for you. Forgive again and again until the pain is history. The most powerful tool of forgiveness I have found is the following ritual from the indigenous wisdom of Hawaii.

Ho'oponopono: 'The Clearing'

I used this ritual once in Hawaii when I was about to undergo a *Ha* (breath) ritual, which plunges deep into the subconscious. I was nervous beforehand, wondering what might be in store for me and whether I would feel comfortable releasing it in public. While I was waiting for the session to begin, I picked up a book at random and began to read it. The book was called *Dark Sun, Bright Moon*. It turned out to be a searing account of the brutal treatment of the Native Americans by the white settlers and armies of North America. It told the story of the army general who had cut off the breasts of Native American women and used them for cups; how tribes had been lured into friendship and then wiped out; tales of slaughter and greed that decimated people who had loved and cared for the land that was now 'owned'. I stopped reading, horrified that I was learning all these details for the first time when I was about to go through the profound *Ha* ritual. However, I knew it was not an accident that I should be reading this book at that moment. It reflected my discomfort about the way traditional Hawaiian culture had been almost wiped out by invaders of the past, who have taken control of the islands and 'possess' them in a way that is typical of Western civilization. I was uncomfortable with the knowledge that many of these invaders were *my* people. They came from the culture I was born into. From their prosperity, as they inflicted damage on the earth and the people who cared for it, *I* had benefited.

Taking the responsibility for these actions upon myself, I went out into the forest and murmured the

Ho'oponopono ritual, feeling as I did so a profound release of the guilt and shame I had begun to harbour since my arrival in Hawaii when I learned the details of how its traditional culture had been destroyed. I felt that my sorrow was acknowledged by the ever-present energy within the earth, and replaced with the clear energy that people of my generation can use to make amends.

This is the prayer I used:

Father, Mother, Child as one. If I (name), my family, relatives and ancestors have offended you (name), your family, relatives and ancestors, in thoughts, words, or actions, from the beginning of creation to the present, we humbly, humbly ask your forgiveness. Let this cleanse, purify, release and cut away all the negative memories, blocks, energies and vibrations and transmute these unwanted energies into pure light. As it is said, it is done, and set free.

When you say this prayer, bring the person or people who you want to forgive to mind in front of you, if you cannot work with them in person. Your intention to direct this prayer wholeheartedly to them will have the same effect as if you were holding hands.

Once the prayer is said, let it go. Don't expect a response. If you still feel you need one then say the prayer again, until you expect nothing. Keep releasing, and trust that the release will ultimately bring the response that is needed to resolve the situation. You will know when it has.

Listen: Hear the Music you Make

Understand Your Dreams

Dreams can help you to know yourself in a way that you will find fascinating once you grow familiar with the language your subconscious uses. They incorporate all the paraphernalia of your present life but they are also easy and rewarding reflections of what is deeply important to you, once you get a few rules in hand.

- *Everything in your dream is you.* Even when you are dreaming of loved ones or enemies or colleagues, it is an aspect of yourself in that person that you are dreaming about.
- *The way you felt about what was happening* is the most important aspect of your dream. The dream is a helpful reflection of your deepest feelings, which you may not have been giving yourself permission to feel in your daily life.
- *You are the expert in what the symbols in your dream mean* – no matter how distant cultures such as the Mayans, or the Cherokee or the Zulus may have interpreted the signs in your dreams. The interpretations of various cultures may have been a part of your experience or your education and this could be significant. But in the final analysis it is you who is the expert in your own consciousness and you need to search your mind to ask why a particular symbol or sign is important to you. To do this, any book of information can be helpful, especially a

good dictionary or encyclopaedia. When you read the definition or description of what you have dreamed you will recognize how it relates to you.

If your dreams are going to be helpful in guiding you through your life then the first thing you have to do, of course, is to remember them. If you have been having nightmares then you'll have no trouble remembering them. Nightmares indicate that there is a critical situation in your life that you need to pay attention to. Other dreams may be helpful and encouraging as you move through the milestones in your life – if you take the trouble to remember them and note them down. Remembering dreams gets easier once you begin to understand their language, but the best way to start is to keep a scrap notebook and a pen beside your bed and scribble down your dream as soon as you wake up. If you can't get time to write it down, tell someone your dream. Once you put the dream into words it will clarify it and the events will become 'real' enough to remember.

If you can't do this, or have trouble remembering your dream even when you have just come out of it, close your eyes at some point during the day and take yourself back to the most significant aspect of it that sticks in your mind. When you have this in your mind's eye, look around and see if there was anyone else you were aware of sharing your dream with, any type of movement or colours that you can remember, and above all, how you felt about being in the situation you found yourself in.

It doesn't matter whether you understand your dream or not when you note it down. Often you will be astonished when you look back at these scribbled notes to see how much your subconscious understood about what was going to happen in your life while you weren't consciously aware of it. You will begin to see how your dreams can guide you forward, and your own subconscious is directing you to pursue choices that make you happier and healthier

How Do You Talk to Yourself?

The tool that turns thought into a tangible force is usually a word. Without words, thought vanishes into the continuous round of energy in the universe, unless expressed in music or images. Many of us keep up a continuous silent commentary on our actions, sometimes even speaking it out loud. But how do you talk to yourself? Do you praise your efforts, or are you always self-critical? If you were a small child and an adult talked to you in this way, how would you respond? Children respond better to encouragement than to criticism, and yet we often subject the vulnerable uncertain 'child' in ourselves to a barrage of hostile commentary more severe than any we would impose on someone else. The best way to understand how you speak to yourself is to go on a diet. Not a normal kind of diet. It only lasts a week and you can eat what you like. But this diet will shine a light on your internal conversation.

The Happiness Diet

The rules are very simple, but you must follow them to the letter.

- The first day you are allowed three negative statements about yourself.
- The second day you are allowed two negative statements about yourself.
- The third day you are allowed one.
- For the rest of the week you are allowed none at all. Every time a negative thought about your abilities or your achievements comes up in your mind, catch it and transform it into a positive statement. For example, instead of saying to yourself, 'I can't swim', you can say, 'I am learning how to swim. I haven't succeeded yet but whatever is possible for another human being is possible for me.'

At the end of a week you will have a clear idea of the blocks you habitually put in your way. You may hear the language of a parent or teacher echoing in the words you have used to limit yourself, and so you may understand why you have chosen to do so in the past.

Desire: Have What You Want

Creating change demands that you use your will to bring about your desire. The power of imagining your desires cannot be overstated. Desire is your creative strength. It is creative not just for you, but for your family, your society and for the whole planet. It is what propels us forward. New generations, homes, houses, new technologies are all born out of the creative will that comes from our imagination combined with desire. So desire actually creates the reality we live in, as individuals and as a society.

We have been taught to repress our desires as individuals, from the most fundamental sexual level to the desire to create something different from the environment we have grown up in. Society has found the desires of individuals threatening, while actually thriving and changing because of the desires being expressed and pursued. So we have tended not to recognize the beauty of this creative power within us.

When we want something that is not in conflict with someone else's desire, there is nothing to stop us having it. This works because our most fundamental desire as human beings is for love – to love and be loved, even though in some individuals this desire is converted into fear of not being loved and replaced with the desire for power.

The exercises you have done so far may seem to be passive in nature, but in fact you have been removing impediments to this powerful creative force in you. Your desire *is* the power of attraction you embody, but in order for you to bring it into being you need to make sure that there is no conflicting force to interfere with it. Conflict can come from outside. Everyone's desire has equal weight. More usually, though, conflict comes from within. You prevent yourself from having what you want. When you become aware of your internal conversation and the reasons why it has taken the form that it has, you give yourself the opportunity to change it and focus your energy on what makes you happy.

There is no way to happiness. Happiness is the way.

Buddha

You are meant to be happy. To understand the importance of taking what you need to express what you want, picture this. You see a beautiful rose. Nearby there is a lovely apple tree, spreading its branches, laden with sweet apples. Would you look at the tree and wish it had fewer apples and took less from the soil, so the rose could have more flowers? It doesn't make sense. You would want each plant to take everything it needs to show the full beauty of its form according to its nature.

Isn't this what you want for yourself? In times of hardship, parents want to ensure that their children survive, even if this means they must deny themselves. Yet for most of us, most of the time, self-denial is an unnecessary habit that undermines our joy in life.

Great desire demands great will, and when you sharpen your will with the clear image of your desire, you achieve results beyond your understanding.

Healing Illness

If you have a potentially fatal illness then there is no doubt about what you desire. Your hopes are crystallized in the desire to overcome the illness and live. The clarity of this desire can galvanize your will. That's why so many people who have had a serious illness or a near-death experience say it has taught them how to live and be happy – as it did me. As well as the changes you put in place to make your life the one you want to live, you will need to use your will to change what is happening in your body.

- Make yourself a contract to dedicate time to healing your body, no matter how you are feeling on any day. Give yourself a time frame of weeks or months, by the end of which you expect to see physical evidence of this healing.
- Allocate yourself three periods of 10–20 minutes each day when you can be quiet and undisturbed and focus entirely on your healing.
- At the start of each period, sit down and close your eyes. Release your breath, letting your diaphragm collapse, telling yourself to relax. Do this three times, and then count down from 10 to 1. You are now in a space where your mind can create any dream you choose.
- Focus on what is wrong. Send your 'agents' to dissolve a tumour, release a blockage, revivify a damaged organ – whatever it is that your body needs. Your 'agents' can be anything that you truly believe in, and will be as individual as you are.

- Imagine the situation you desire, as vividly and completely as if you were creating it for a film. See this scene evolving from the current situation.

- Persist with this image patiently and consistently every day until you see results. Make it as realistic as you can, so that you can feel the effect that success has on you. The feeling is most important. Allow yourself to be confident of success in this special time, even if you have doubts at other times and other people in your life call this a false dream. When people talk about 'false hope', they underestimate the power we have to create new realities in our lives. Allow yourself to dream, however unlikely it may sometimes seem. You are unleashing the creative power of your mind to heal your body.

- Maintain this programme alongside any medical treatment you are having. Make the most of medical interventions you have chosen by seeing them as assisting you in this process, rather than invasive or destructive.

- Persist and be patient with yourself when there are setbacks. You will be astonished by the power of your positive mind.

Find Your Happiness

Many, many people tell me that they don't know what makes them happy. Some people, in fact, unconsciously drive themselves towards disaster in order to find a place where they will be forced to reach out for survival and happiness. This may happen, but self-destructive behaviour can create a reality that you 'believe' in, just as positive behaviour does. To recover from self-destruction you need to show yourself that you can create your reality by setting yourself some positive goals that you can achieve.

Desires that make you happy are expressed more often in the language of your body than the language of your mind. They start with the things that your hands love to do, the sounds, the tastes and the sensations that you enjoy, the environment that makes you relaxed, the people you want to be with. Then, they are the situation that makes this possible, the loving relationships you can create or the secure home where you can enjoy these things. Your desires may seem to be in conflict with what you have believed to be possible, but leave your beliefs aside for the present. You will never be happy until you acknowledge your desires and find a way to pursue them. Listen to what feels good and you will know what they are. If it's been a long time since you even asked for something you want for your birthday, this following exercise will sort out your goals.

Signposts

- Make a chart as shown overleaf on a sheet of paper. Put the date at the top. It's a date you will want to remember.
- Write the heading of these important parts of your life in the left-hand column. Arrange them on the basis of how important they are to you, with the most important first. Now score each one on how satisfactory you feel it is in your life

at present, with 10 as most satisfactory and 1 as
least.

- Next to that score, write a sentence or a phrase
  that you think honestly describes the way you
  feel about the current state of affairs.

A sample chart is shown opposite.

This exercise will give you a clear idea of what you
tell yourself about what is important to you in your
life. Read what you have written and see if it accurately
reflects what you say to yourself about these aspects of
daily living.

Put the paper away until the next day and then . . .

- Look again at the words you have used to describe
  your current situation. How would you change
  these if you were describing your dreams? Reword
  your description as if it described the best outcome
  you can imagine. Let your sentence express in the
  present how it *feels* to have succeeded in your aim.
- Make the statements for your new situation
  simple but as ambitious as you can. Dare to
  name your dreams. How else will you achieve
  them? Allow your language to go beyond any
  habitual limitations. An ancient yogic exercise for
  developing the different capacities of the brain has
  this as an example – to develop your artistic ability
  it recommends that you repeat this statement to
  yourself: 'I am originality. The fountain of creative
  ability springs from within me, because I am one

Sample Chart

Health: physical issues including weight, eyesight	4	I am overweight and I can't stop eating	
Security: job; money; home	3	I don't like my job but I need the money	
Romantic relationship: sex; communication; companionship	5	I love my partner but we argue constantly	
Family relationships: parents, siblings, children			
Social interaction: friends, community, colleagues			
Creative self-expression: art; writing; gardening; music			
Sense of mission or purpose in your life			
Spiritual guidance/support			

with Nature's artist. Nothing is beyond my powers. I can paint, draw, sing, etc. exceedingly well.'

- Rescore with a mark that says how much it will mean to you when this dream is a tangible reality. 10 is ecstatic; 1 means you don't care.

A chart showing further detail is shown opposite.

Make the signposts with the biggest difference in numbers between the first and second score your top priority for treatment as follows:

- Repeat your dream statements every day in different ways: write them on cards where you can see and read them, go over them in your mind in the morning, or say them to yourself as you go to sleep at night.
- Don't be intimidated if you feel that they are far from the 'truth'.
- Repeat them until you have covered everything on the list.
- When you have written the new patterns of thinking on your sheet of paper and copied them onto cards or perhaps onto your PC or phone, do one more thing with this paper. Hide it. Put it somewhere like the back of a drawer or inside the flap of a book where you are likely to forget about it. If you come across it in a few years' time, you will be astonished by the progress you have made.

Focus on what you want. Enjoy what you have. Accept what you get.

Health: physical issues including weight, eyesight	4	I am overweight and I can't stop eating	8	I am slim and strong and I enjoy every bite of food I eat.
Security: job; money; home	3	I don't like my job but I need the money	9	Money comes to me from doing what I love to do. I would do it anyway even if I didn't get paid. All my needs are taken care of.
Romantic relationship: sex; communication; companionship	5	I love my partner but we argue constantly	10	I love my partner the way he/she is and I see that our differences from each other create a strong balanced unit where we are both free and secure.
Family relationships: parents, siblings, children				
Social interaction: friends, community, colleagues				
Creative self-expression: art; writing; gardening; music				
Sense of mission or purpose in your life				
Spiritual guidance/support				

Prayer

We must feel the feeling as if the prayer has already been answered.

Tibetan abbot

What you have been doing is effectively a prayer, though you may not recognize it as such. Prayer is something so simple, so familiar to every culture since the beginning of records, that we think we know all about it, but there are plenty of misconceptions.

A prayer can have magical effect. So we need to do it. Almost everything in this book is about the power that you have to help yourself. But the greatest help you can give yourself is to ask for help. When you do that sincerely, you discover power beyond your limits: your invisible giant.

What stands between us and the help we need is our pride. We feel responsible for managing everything. The more unsure of ourselves we are, the more we focus on our differences from others. We judge other people as greater or lesser than us and find no common ground. Even in our misery, we think that we are special, incomprehensible. We cling to a notion of separate identity, our 'ego'. Sometimes the self-identity you have grown used to feels like the only thing you have left to defend yourself with, even if you don't like it. To let it go feels like a kind of death, even while it is pushing you to a sense of separation that feels like a void.

Prayer comes at the moment when you breach that separation. Out of desperation or belief you open up to the power of your environment. Your small self within the grand scale of nature humbles you – you see your weakness. In the act of asking for help, you are opening your heart to gratitude. Once you open up, help comes to you.

Choosing to pray is the creative choice of your life. You go beyond your sense of separation, and you discover that the great power that imbues everything in the world responds to you when you ask it to. Truth is always a paradox. The paradox of prayer is that the more you are aware of your small place in the universe, the more the universe seems to notice you and give you what makes you happy.

Prayer takes many forms. You must find the language that resonates with you.

Three Styles of Prayer

- Many religious schools paint elaborate verbal and visual pictures of the gods in their prayers. In Hinduism and Buddhism the gods are aspects of the universal consciousness. The prayer conjures their essence in detail so that you elevate your focus to the pure form of consciousness they embody. A Tibetan Buddhist prayer to the Medicine Buddha, for example, describes every aspect of his appearance and his environment, and the student of this prayer learns the symbolic significance of every object he has about him. The prayer is a long rhythmic recitation of his attributes, so that you conjure his capacity to heal as visually and tangibly real when you pray to him. Then you can merge yourself with this image of healing bounty. You take the Medicine Buddha's healing power into your consciousness. This healing becomes part of your thought. You absorb it. You own it, and the image has given you its strength.

- Hawaiian religious teachers were called *kahuna* – keepers of the secret. They used to pray in a similar way: long recitative prayers, describing each attribute of the gods, their heritage and relationship to each other and to the person praying. The prayer rooted the supplicant in the environment, calling on the ancestors who had learned their powers from the gods who created the land and sea. Sometimes these prayers would take days to recite and many years to learn. The process of chanting them conjured an intensity of feeling that overcame material limitations. There are abundant stories of Hawaiian *kahuna* who could perform 'instant' healing, and walk unscathed over hot lava. When the Christian missionaries came to Hawaii, the *kahuna* were outlawed. Many of them eventually adapted their spiritual tradition to Christianity. They became Christian priests and converted the traditional prayers to a simpler form of expression. They summarized the spirit in the word 'aloha': love. In their prayers they called on the power of the superconscious, God, to come to the help of the Mother (logical mind) and Child (emotional and physical mind) in humanity. They achieved powerful results with the new prayers, as they had with the old ones. One of these initiated Hawaiian priests, David Kaonohiokala Bray, described this transition as moving from the dark (old) way of prayer to the light (new) way.

- In 1989 the Chinese Qi Gong healers of the medicine-less hospital near Beijing made a video of healers working on a woman with a cancerous tumour in her bladder. They put an ultrasound scan on her stomach so that they could track the progress of the tumour as they healed it. While three healers chant over the patient with gathering intensity, the ultrasound image shows the tumour shrinking before our eyes. So what is the prayer the healers are chanting as they create this extraordinary effect? They are not praying to any Western idea of God as such, but trusting themselves to the universal *chi* that pervades everything. Using their minds and imaginations to see material reality as they wish it to be, rather than as it has appeared, they chant over and over again: 'Mayo le. Mayo le.' The words mean: 'It never was. It never was.' As they chant, the tumour becomes invisible.

You do need conviction to utter a prayer, but it can be the conviction of hope rather than knowledge of what will come in response to you. Some people want to know exactly what will happen and how if they pray, but you need to pray with an open mind. Only then can you receive a response which is bigger than any you could have imagined for yourself.

Prayer can be effective in any form, in any environment, in any language, aimed at any power. What is important is the feeling you speak it with. Be sure to visualize and feel the power you are praying to. Speak your prayer with humility, appealing to a power that you know is greater than yourself, whether it be the power of god, of the earth, of the moon and stars, the power of angels or super-terrestrial beings. Say your prayer with the sincerity of an open heart. It will be answered in ways that surprise you.

Pray out loud, committing your whole body and mind to the essence of your prayer. Pray in the language of your heart, the one that resonates with your deepest feelings. Use that language in the way that speaks most directly to you. This will be more powerful than any prayer that you have learned. Some prayers are in unfamiliar languages, like Sanskrit or Tibetan, for example. The sound of the language has a vibration that has a powerful impact. Even so, pray in your native language also, until you are confident that the prayer you utter truly captures your feelings.

As you speak, see and feel the result of the prayer in your imagination. Let yourself imagine it intensely as though it had already happened.

Finally, trust your prayer. Once you have delivered it, let it go. A prayer is not a replacement for your efforts but a profound support to them. Concentrate on what you can do and let greater powers take care of the rest. Extraordinary things are within your reach. Trust yourself to achieve them.

Resources

WEBSITES

www.annaparkinson.com
www.healer.ch
www.sacredhealer.co.uk

BOOKS

Healing

Brofman, Martin, *Anything Can be Healed*, Findhorn Press, 2003

Brofman, Martin, *Improve your Vision*, Findhorn Press, 2004

Davies, Dr Brenda, *The Rainbow Journey: Seven Steps to Self Healing*, Coronet, 1999

Emoto, Masuru (IHM General Research Institute), *Messages from Water*, HADO Publishing, 1999

Jim, Kahuna Harry Uhane and Garnette Arledge, *Wise Secrets of Aloha*, Weiser Books, 2007

Murphy, Joseph, *The Power of your Subconscious Mind*, Prentice Hall, 1963

Shattock, E H, *Mind your Body*, Turnstone Books, 1979

Science

Chopra, Deepak, *Quantum Healing*, Bantam, 1989

Lipton, Bruce, *The Biology of Belief*, Hay House, 2005

McTaggart, Lynn, *The Field*, HarperCollins, 2001

Orzel, Chad, *How to Teach Quantum Physics to your Dog*, Oneworld Publications, 2010

Pert, Dr Candace, *The Molecules of Emotion*, Scribner, 1997

Creativity

Lamott, Anne, *Bird by Bird: Instructions on Writing and Life*, Anchor Books, 2007

Yoga and the Yogi science of Breathing

Avalon, Arthur, tr., *The Serpent Power*, Dover Publications, 1974

Desikachar, T K V, *The Heart of Yoga, Developing a Personal Practice*, Inner Traditions International, 1995

Iyengar, B K S, *Light on Yoga*, George Allen & Unwin, 1966

Also by Anna Parkinson

Nature's Alchemist: John Parkinson, Herbalist to Charles I, Frances Lincoln, 2007